Anatomy of the Eyelid, Orbit, and Lacrimal System

Edward H. Bedrossian, Jr • Richard R. Schmidt
Robert C. Della Rocca • Bradley N. Lemke
Editors

Anatomy of the Eyelid, Orbit, and Lacrimal System

A Dissection Manual

Springer

Editors
Edward H. Bedrossian, Jr, MD, FACS
Wills Eye Hospital
Philadelphia, PA, USA

Robert C. Della Rocca, MD, FACS
Ichahn School of Medicine
New York Eye and Ear Infirmary
New York, NY, USA

Richard R. Schmidt, PhD
Sydney Kimmel Medical College
Thomas Jefferson University
Philadelphia, PA, USA

Bradley N. Lemke, MD, FACS
School of Medicine and Public Health
University of Wisconsin System
Madison, WI, USA

ISBN 978-3-030-88264-8 ISBN 978-3-030-88265-5 (eBook)
https://doi.org/10.1007/978-3-030-88265-5

This Springer imprint is published by the registered company Springer Nature Switzerland AG
The registered company address is: Gewerbestrasse 11, 6330 Cham, Switzerland

I owe an unimaginable amount of gratitude to my best friend and wife, Dulcie, for her never-ending support and encouragement for this work and throughout my career. All of my children, Allison, Garret, Robert, and Ryan, and their spouses, Jon, Katie, Ashley, and Lisa, are more than deserving of considerable praise and thanks for their patience, understanding, and continued support over the years. The final portion of this dedication is to our seven grandchildren, Jack, Sofia, Lizzie, Ella, Bryson, Joie, and Matthew, as well as to my present and former students who have made this educational experience remarkably fulfilling.

Richard R. Schmidt, PhD

To my wife Iryna and daughter Olesya for their ever-present love and support.

To my extended family at Wills Eye Hospital and Temple Ophthalmology Department , for their dedication to excellence in patient care, resident education, and research.

Edward H. Bedrossian, Jr, MD, FACS

I wish to express gratitude to my ever-supportive wife Gale and loving family, and I thank Richard K Dortzbach, MD and Orkan George Stasior, MD for sharing with me their passion for the anatomy.

Bradley N. Lemke, MD, FACS

Preface

A strong foundation in anatomy is the basis for excellence in surgery. There are many outstanding textbooks on anatomy of the eyelids, orbit, and lacrimal System. This textbook, however, is different in that it presents a step-by-step dissection in a layered approach, simplifying the overwhelmingly complex anatomy.

Not all structures will be clearly evident in all specimens. Therefore, sharing of well dissected structures with others is encouraged. The dissection is best performed slowly and carefully to limit accidental damage to underlying structures. A basic knowledge of the anatomy prior to the dissection will enhance the experience and allow for a better three-dimensional appreciation.

The manual consists of seven chapters. To maximize the use of each specimen, it is recommended to follow the chapters sequentially. Chapter 1 describes how the specimens are prepared and stored. Chapter 2 describes dissection of the eyelids. Chapter 3 describes dissection of the anterior orbit, posterior to the orbital septum. Chapter 4 demonstrates the cavernous sinus. Chapters 5 and 6 describe the dissection of the orbit from above and from a lateral approach, respectively. Finally , Chapter 7 demonstrates the nasolacrimal system and paranasal sinuses.

This "dissection manual" has been in the making since 1983, when Edward H. Bedrossian Jr., finished his ophthalmic plastic and reconstructive surgery fellowship with Bryon Smith, John Simonton, and Robert Della Rocca. As a fellow, he met Dr Bradley Lemke where a respected friendship developed over a common interest in orbital and facial anatomy. With a strong foundation in three-dimensional anatomy, Dr Bedrossian joined the Oculoplastic and Reconstructive Surgery Department at Wills Eye Hospital. In 1984, he became the director of the Annual Wills Eye Hospital Resident Orbital Dissection Course. He met Richard R. Schmidt, then Associate Professor of Anatomy, Pathology, and Cell Biology at Thomas Jefferson University College of Medicine. Over the next 38 years, without interruption, the two developed and refined an instructional course that is regarded by residents at Wills Eye Hospital as one of the most important courses of their residency. It expanded to include ophthalmology residents at Temple University and Philadelphia College of Osteopathic Medicine. Over 700 residents and oculofacial plastic fellows have benefited from the course, which follows the step-by-step approach outlined in this manual.

Philadelphia, PA, USA — Edward H. Bedrossian, Jr, MD, FACS
Richard R. Schmidt, PhD
New York, NY, USA — Robert C. Della Rocca, MD, FACS
Madison, WI, USA — Bradley N. Lemke, MD, FACS

Acknowledgments

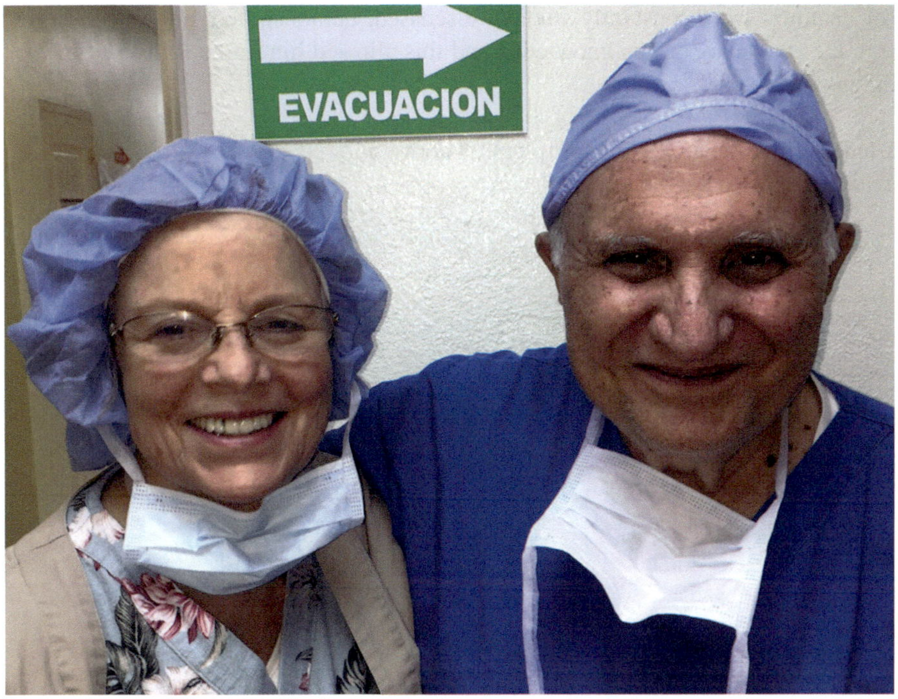

An atlas of this nature is the result of the persistent efforts of many. We are grateful to Dr. Robert Della Rocca for his inspiration, example, and support throughout the process. Unfortunately, he passed away shortly before the text was published and did not see the final version. Below is a memorial tribute to him co-written by his dedicated and loving wife, Darlene and son, David. We appreciate Bradley N. Lemke for his consultative contribution and expertise. We thank our colleagues at Wills Eye Hospital who have assisted with lectures and teaching at the dissections. We appreciate the assistance of Philip (Chris) Marcucci, the Dissection Facility Coordinator at Sidney Kimmel Medical College of Thomas Jefferson University, for his help in procurement and preparation of specimens under Dr. Schmidt's supervision.

The authors wish to thank Alessanda Intili , who as a third-year ophthalmology resident dedicated countless hours in the laboratory performing the dissections and photographing various steps. We are equally appreciative of Mr. Jack Scully, in the photography department at Wills Eye Hospital.

The authors are indebted to the professionals at Springer, especially Asja Rehse (Editor, Clinical Medicine) and Lee Klein (Senior Editor, Atlases), for their enthusiasm in bringing this atlas to completion.

We acknowledge and celebrate the life of Robert C. Della Rocca, MD, who served as a leader in his field of oculoplastic and orbital surgery. Dr. Della Rocca was the son of immigrant parents and grew up in New York City surrounded by a loving family. In the course of his career as a student, physician, and surgeon, he travelled from The Bronx, Omaha, Vietnam, and back to New York City. In this period, he served as Captain and Battalion Surgeon in the US Army, Chief Resident at the New York Eye and Ear Infirmary, and Section Chief of Oculoplastic Surgery at the Mount Sinai Health System.

Dr. Della Rocca was a determined and steadfast clinician and surgeon through his career. He recognized that an intimate knowledge of anatomy allowed him to be effective in accomplishing the highest level of care that he saw as necessary. Dr. Della Rocca's greatest passion was serving as a teacher to his residents and fellows throughout his career. The clinical applications of anatomy were constantly studied, discussed, demonstrated, and utilized. He found refuge in the constancy of this knowledge and this allowed him to be fulfilled as a mentor to generations of doctors.

Darlene Della Rocca, MD, FACS (pictured above with Dr Robert Della Rocca)
David A. Della Rocca, MD (son)

Contents

Contributors

Edward H. Bedrossian, Jr, MD, FACS Wills Eye Hospital, Philadelphia, PA, USA

Richard R. Schmidt, PhD Sydney Kimmel Medical College, Thomas Jefferson University, Philadelphia, PA, USA

Preparation of Specimens for Orbital Dissection Course

1

Richard R. Schmidt

Introduction

The preparation of specimens is a critical component of any orbital dissection course. Thus, the present chapter focuses on the methodology utilized for preparation, subsequent storage, and handling of such specimens.

We routinely harvest undissected or partially dissected heads from embalmed whole-body donations utilized in a variety of undergraduate medical student and allied health student dissection courses. The brains may or may not have been previously removed. In the preparation illustrated below, the brain is present. The ultimate objective is to prepare two quartered orbital specimens from each head such that course participants may have the flexibility of dissecting the eyelids; the orbit from above and below, medially, and laterally; as well as the lacrimal system.

Once the head has been harvested, we typically make all of the required saw cuts on a standard band saw in our dissection facility. The following are the steps for preparing the quartered specimens to be used for the orbital dissection:

1. Proceed by making an axial cut through the upper neck region of the harvested head such that it will sit evenly upright on the saw platform for the initial vertical cut splitting the head into two halves as close to the midline as possible (Fig. 1.1). Be certain to remove any dentures that may be present prior to making this midline cut. The head must be held firmly as this cut is made to ensure that the midline plane is maintained throughout the procedure.

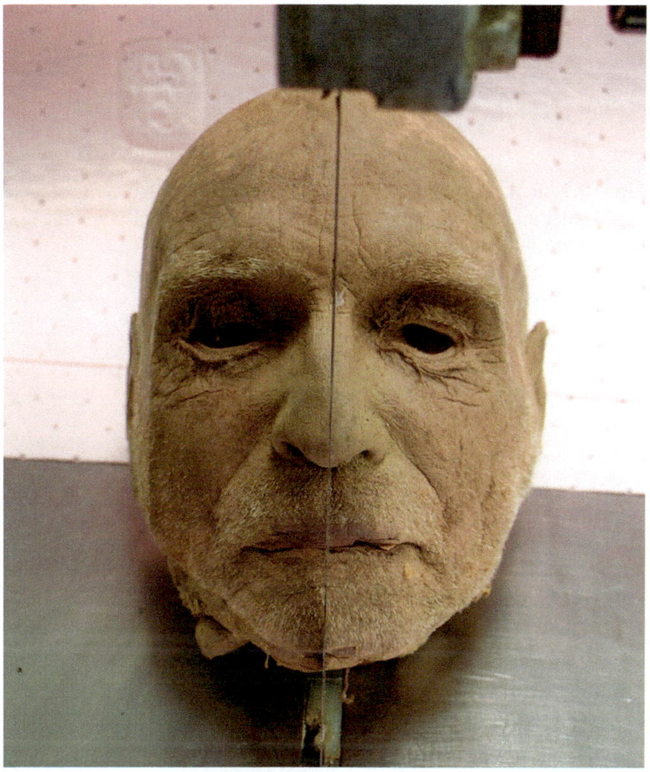

Fig. 1.1 Alignment of initial midline cut

R. R. Schmidt, PhD (✉)
Sydney Kimmel Medical College, Thomas Jefferson University, Philadelphia, PA, USA
e-mail: richard.r.schmidt@jefferson.edu

E. H. Bedrossian, Jr et al. (eds.), *Anatomy of the Eyelid, Orbit, and Lacrimal System*,
https://doi.org/10.1007/978-3-030-88265-5_1

2. Once this midline cut has been completed, the two halves will appear as shown in the lateral view (Fig. 1.2) and a medial view (Fig. 1.3). On the medial aspect of the hemisected head (Fig. 1.3), note the following landmarks: inferior meatus, inferior concha, sphenoid sinus, frontal sinus, corpus callosum, lateral ventricle, cerebellum, and pons.

3. The next step in the preparation process is to make two parallel axial cuts which will result in the quartered orbital specimen. The dotted lines (Fig. 1.4) illustrate the level of each axial cut. The first cut (axial cut A) is typically made slightly above the level of the brow. The second axial cut (axial cut B) is made parallel to the first one, just inferior to the level of the nasal spine.

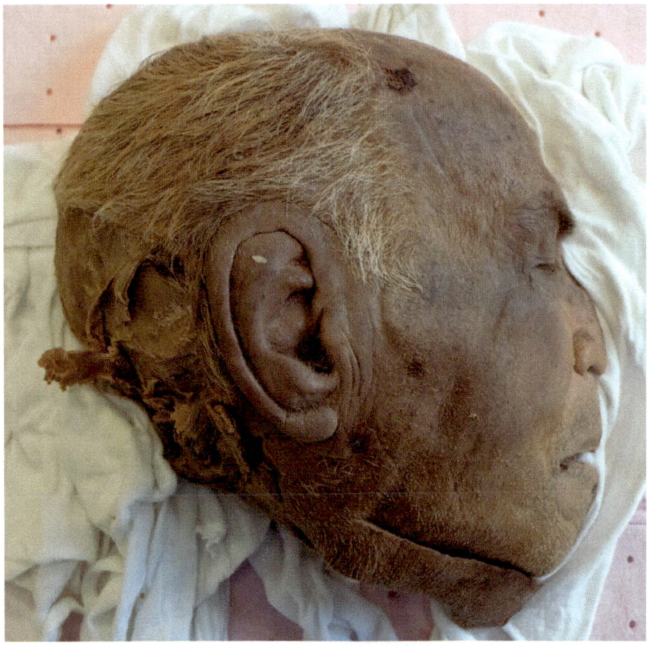

Fig. 1.2 Lateral aspect of hemisected head

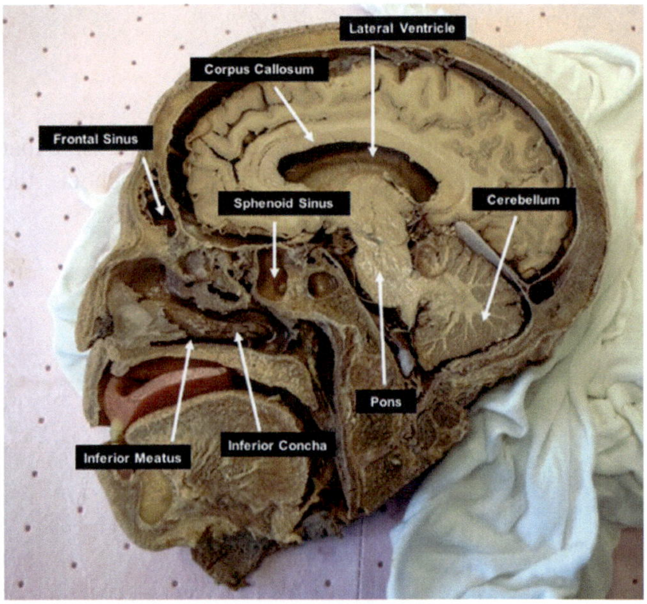

Fig. 1.3 Medial aspect of hemisected head with landmarks

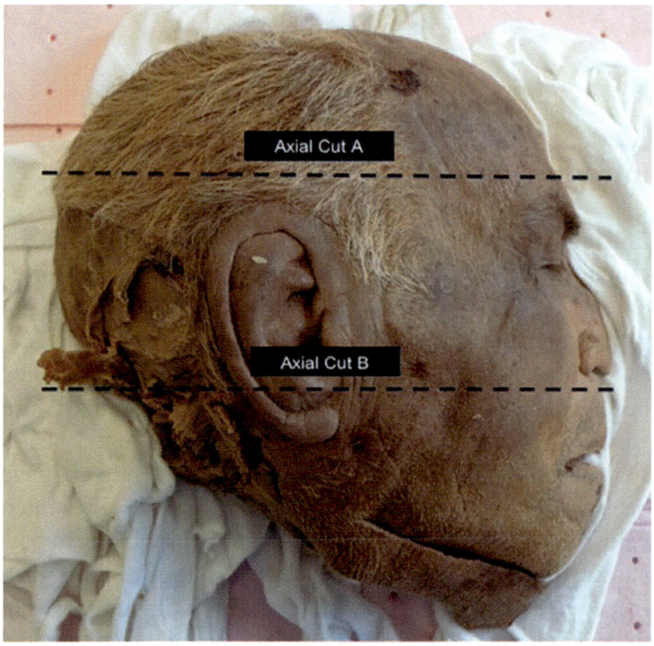

Fig. 1.4 Lateral aspect of hemisected head illustrating the positioning for axial cuts (a) and (b)

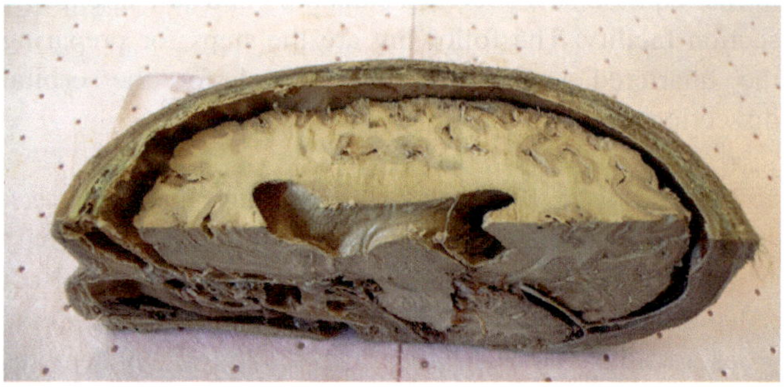

Fig. 1.5 Superomedial view of quartered orbital specimen

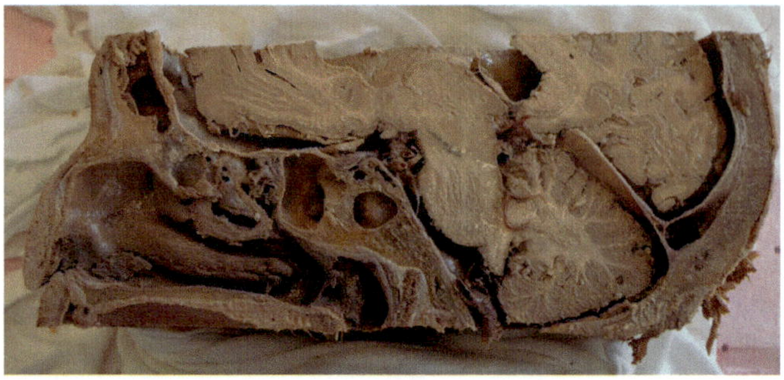

Fig. 1.6 Medial aspect of quartered orbital specimen

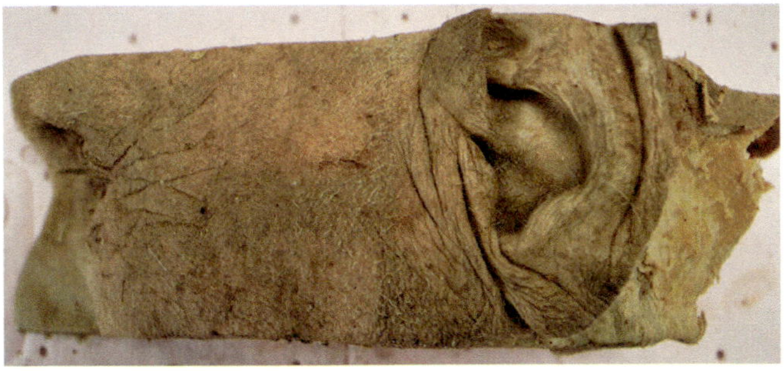

Fig. 1.7 Lateral aspect of quartered orbital specimen

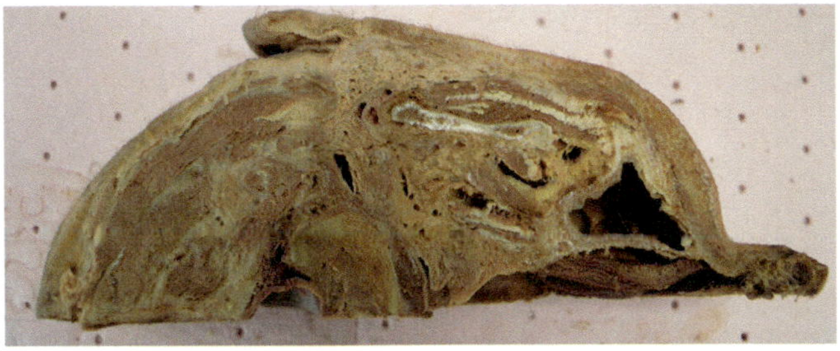

Fig. 1.8 Inferior aspect of quartered orbital specimen

4. Once the two parallel axial cuts have been made as outlined in step 3 above, the quartered orbital specimen is examined from four different vantage points. The superomedial aspect (Fig. 1.5), the medial aspect (Fig. 1.6), the lateral aspect (Fig. 1.7), and the inferior aspect (Fig. 1.8) of the quartered orbital specimen are examined.
5. Once the quartered orbital specimens have been prepared, they are wrapped in cloth toweling, soaked in a diluted holding solution, and placed in a 5-gallon container filled with sufficient holding solution to cover the specimens. The container with the specimens is placed in a cold room until needed for the course.
6. Two or possibly three participants for each specimen are advised to maximize the learning experience. On the day of the course, each pair of participants receives one quartered orbital specimen on a stainless steel tray together

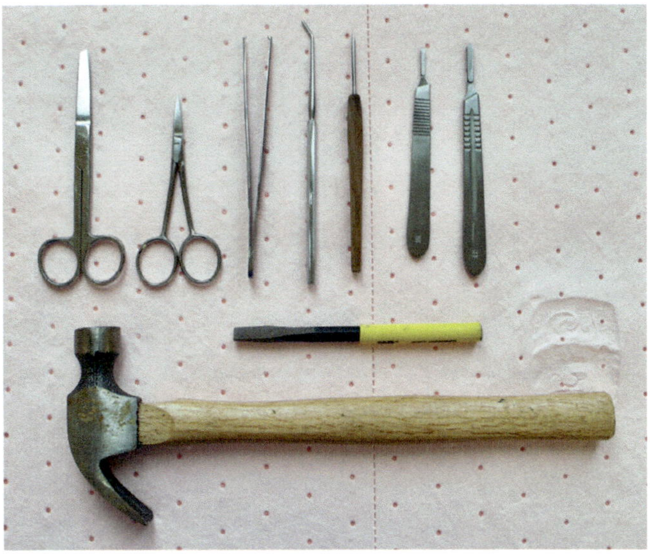

Fig. 1.9 Instrument set with which to perform orbital dissections

with the instruments (Fig. 1.9) with which to perform their dissections. They include an osteotome and mallet, Stevens scissors, probes, forceps, blade handles, and #10, #11, and #15 blades.
7. Specimens are wrapped with cloth toweling and soaked in holding solution, between dissection sessions. The most efficient use of the specimen is to first dissect the eyelids, then the orbit, and finally the lacrimal drainage system.

Suggested Reading

Kakizaki H, Lay-Leng S, Asamoto K, Nakano T, Selva D, Leibovitch I. Dissection of the eyelid and orbit with modernised anatomical findings. The Open Anatomy Journal. 2010;2:5–24.

Laurenson RD. Dissection of the Orbit. The Anatomical Record. 1965;152(4):537–9.

Rosse C, Gaddum-Rosse P. Textbook of anatomy. Philadelphia: Lippincott-Raven Publishers; 1997. p. 812–27.

Turvey TA, Golden BA. Orbital anatomy for the surgeon. Oral Maxillofac Surg Clin North Am. 2013;24(4).

The Eyelids

2

Edward H. Bedrossian, Jr

In this chapter, the upper and lower eyelids are dissected in a structurally layered approach, starting anteriorly with the skin and then proceeding posteriorly through the orbicularis oculi muscle and orbital septum to the tarsus. Throughout the dissection, clinical correlation is provided to stress the importance of knowing its anatomy for the management of nonsurgical and surgical conditions.

Skin

1. Make incisions through the skin only, along the lines indicated in Figs. 2.1, 2.2, 2.3, 2.4, 2.5, 2.6, 2.7, and 2.8.

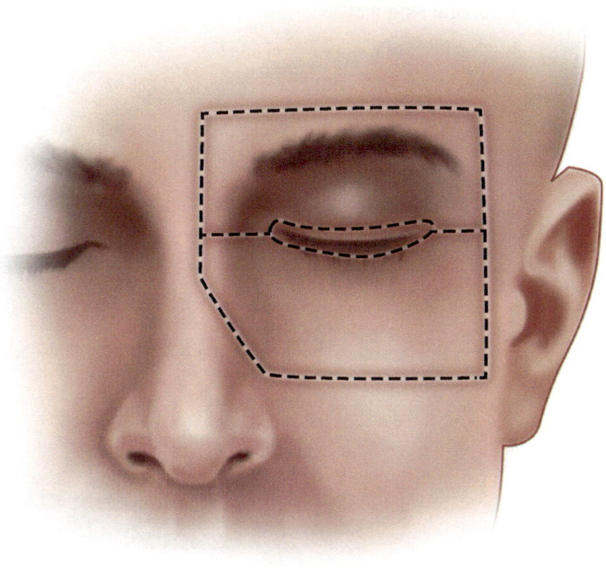

Fig. 2.1 Site for skin incisions

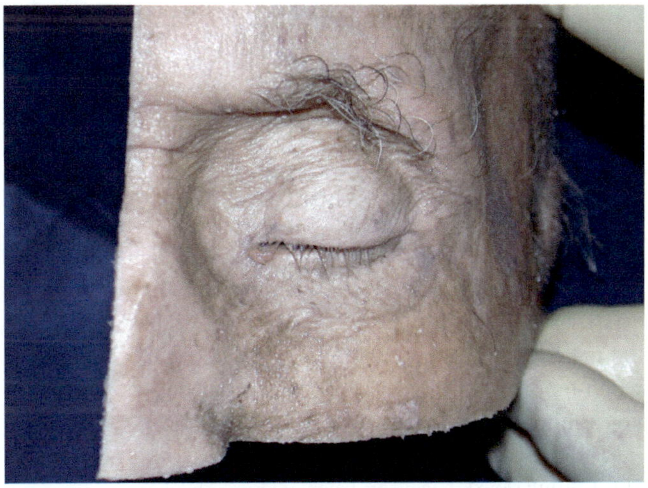

Fig. 2.2 Hemisected specimen, cut above the brow and at lower nares

E. H. Bedrossian, Jr, MD, FACS (✉)
Wills Eye Hospital, Philadelphia, PA, USA

E. H. Bedrossian, Jr et al. (eds.), *Anatomy of the Eyelid, Orbit, and Lacrimal System*,
https://doi.org/10.1007/978-3-030-88265-5_2

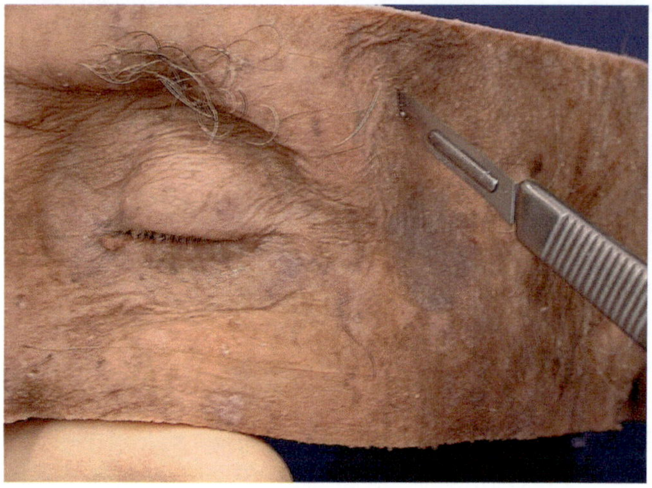

Fig. 2.3 Temporal skin incision

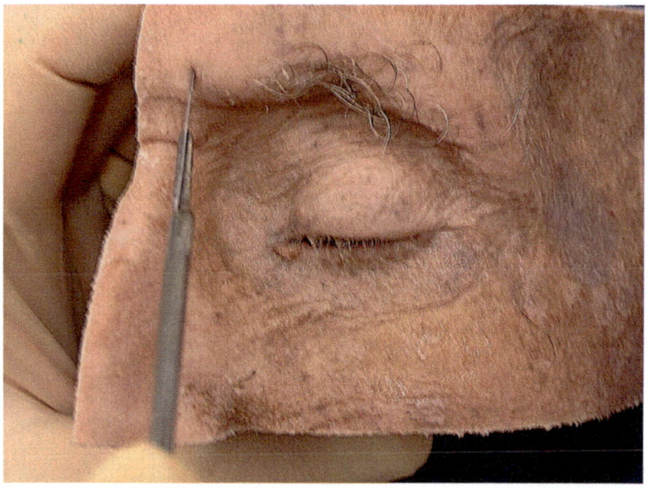

Fig. 2.4 Nasal skin incision

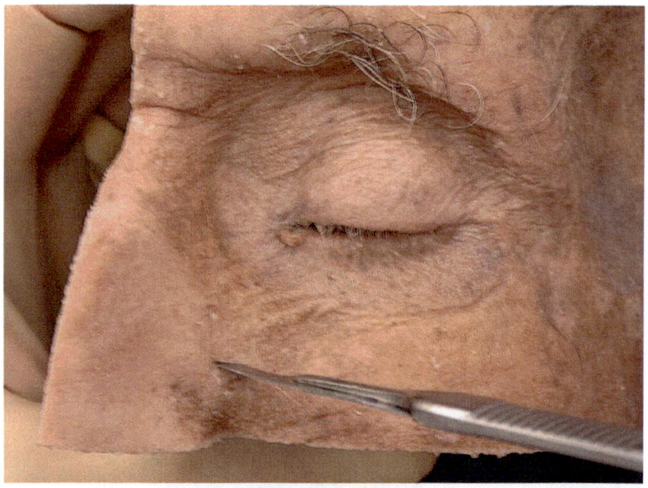

Fig. 2.5 Inferior skin incision, below inferior orbital rim

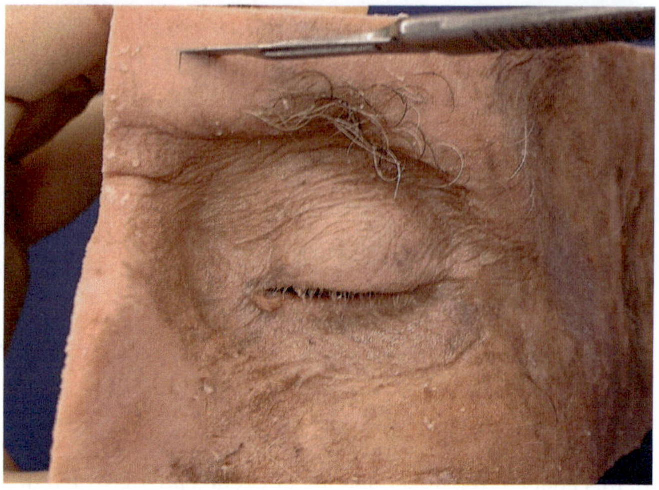

Fig. 2.6 Superior skin incision, above the brow

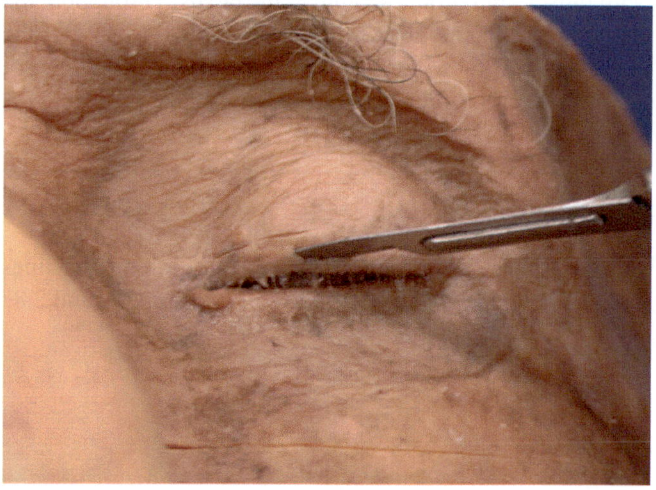

Fig. 2.7 Skin incision along superior eyelid margin

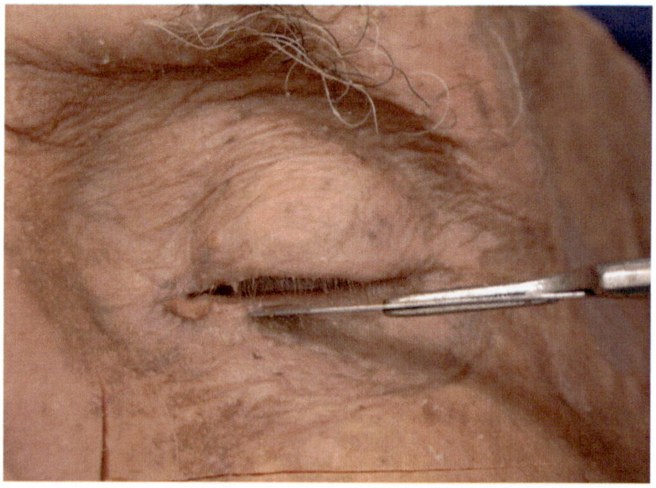

Fig. 2.8 Skin incision along inferior eyelid margin

2. Carefully remove only the skin of the malar region (Figs. 2.9, 2.10, and 2.11), eyelids, and eyebrows (Figs. 2.12 and 2.13).
3. Note the denser skin has denser subcutaneous attachments, particularly the firm attachments over the lateral orbicularis and the medial naso-orbital valley (Fig. 2.12).

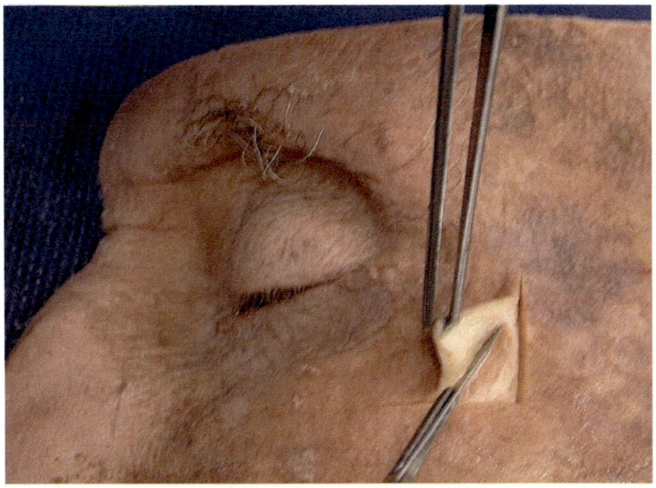

Fig. 2.9 Subcutaneous dissection, temporal malar region

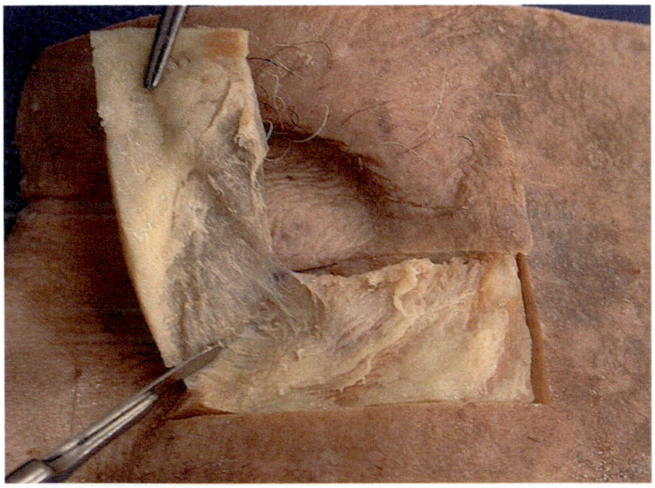

Fig. 2.10 Subcutaneous dissection, nasojugal region, with firm subcutaneous attachments

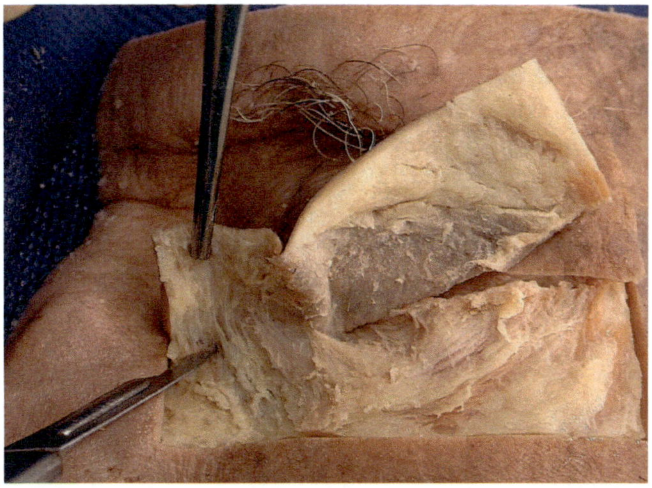

Fig. 2.11 Subcutaneous dissection, nasojugal region, with firm subcutaneous attachments

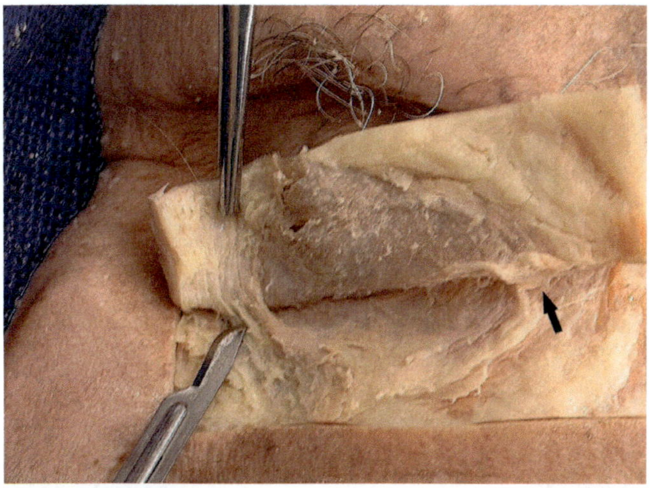

Fig. 2.12 Subcutaneous attachments. Note that the thicker skin has denser subcutaneous attachments especially at the lateral orbicularis oculi (arrow) and medial naso-orbital valley (blade)

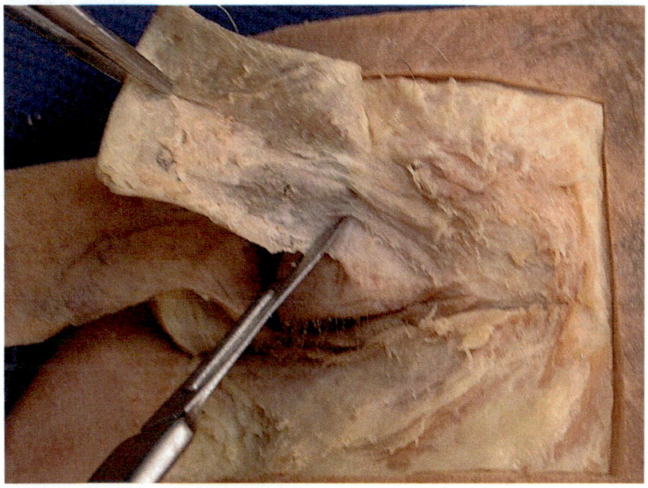

Fig. 2.13 Subcutaneous dissection of the brow and upper eyelid

4. Note the subcutaneous insertion of the corrugator supercilii (Fig. 2.14).
5. Placing the dissected skin flap to the side, note that the thick skin of the temple, eyebrow, glabellar, and malar regions rapidly thins as the eyelids and eyelid margins are approached (Fig. 2.15).

Clinical correlation: Surgical incisions in the thin eyelid skin are not made as "deeply" as those in the thicker skin of the forehead, brow, and malar regions.

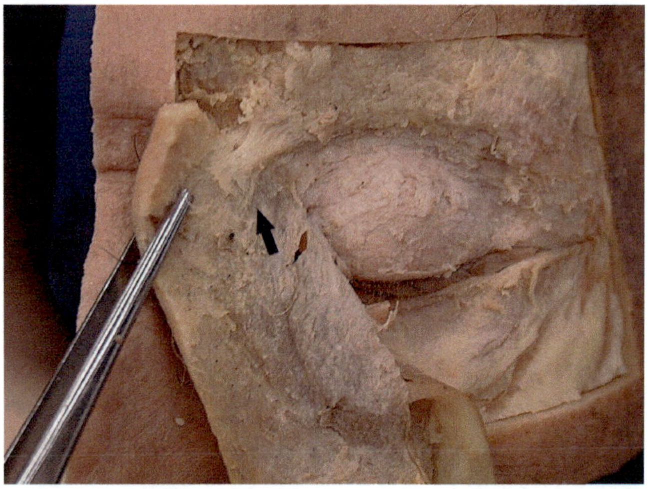

Fig. 2.14 Subcutaneous insertion of the corrugator supercilii muscle (arrow)

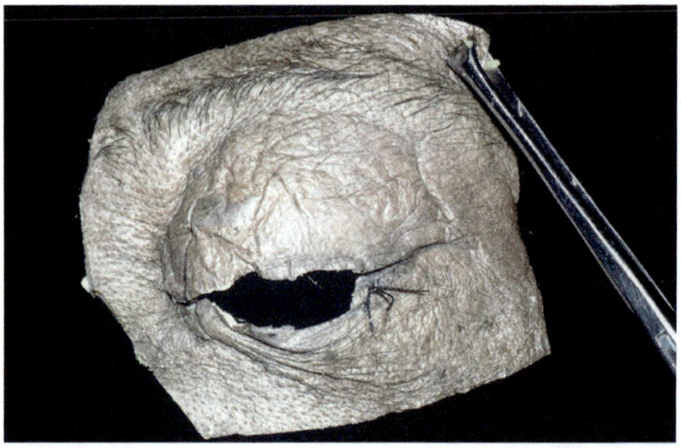

Fig. 2.15 Skin of the brow, eyelids, nasojugal and malar regions, medial canthus, and lateral canthus removed. Note that the thicker skin at the temple, eyebrow, glabellar, and malar regions rapidly thins as the eyelids and eyelid margins are approached

6. Identify the corrugator supercilii near its origin (Fig. 2.16) at the nasal process of the maxillary bone and its subcutaneous insertion (Figs. 2.14 and 2.17) dissected at the medial eyebrow.

Clinical correlation: Site of Botox injections to soften diagonal lines of the glabellar region.

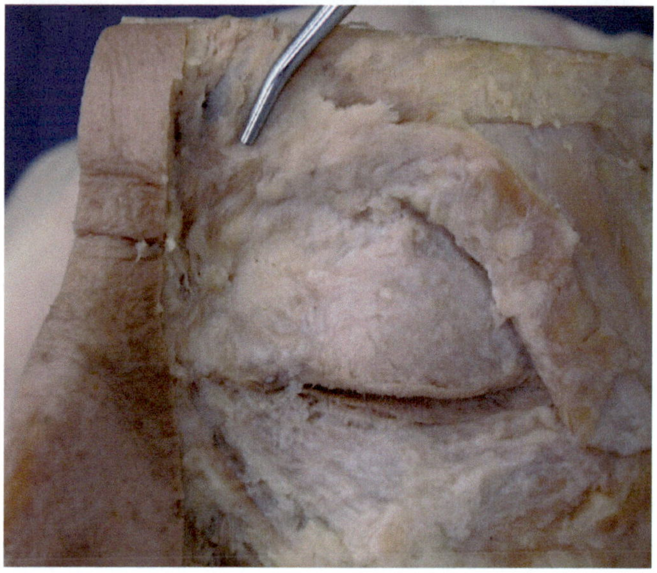

Fig. 2.16 Corrugator supercilii muscle. Pointer near origin at frontal process of maxillary bone

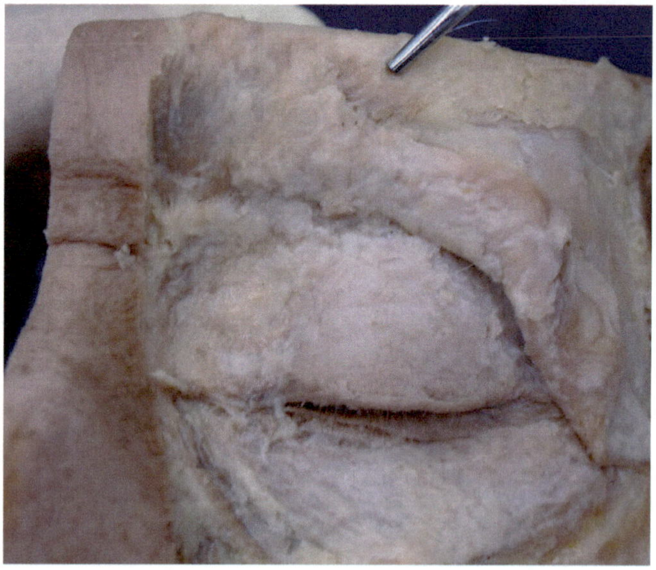

Fig. 2.17 Corrugator supercilii muscle. Pointer in region of subcutaneous insertion at medial brow

Muscle

7. With the skin removed, next clean and expose the underlying orbicularis, frontalis, procerus, levator labii superioris (Fig. 2.18), and levator alae nasae muscles (Fig. 2.19).

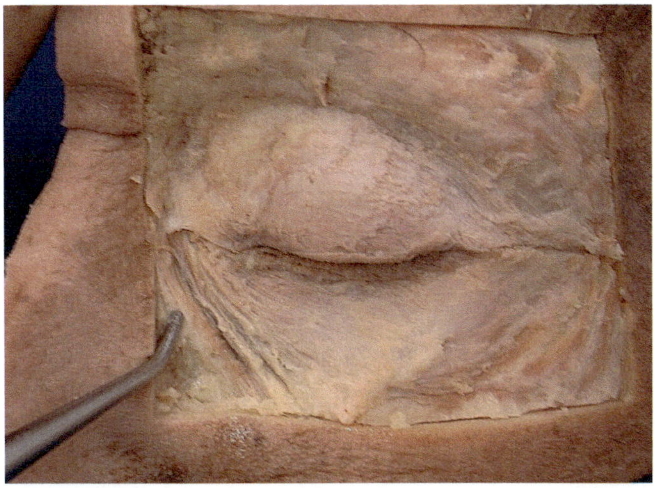

Fig. 2.18 Levator labii superioris muscle at pointer

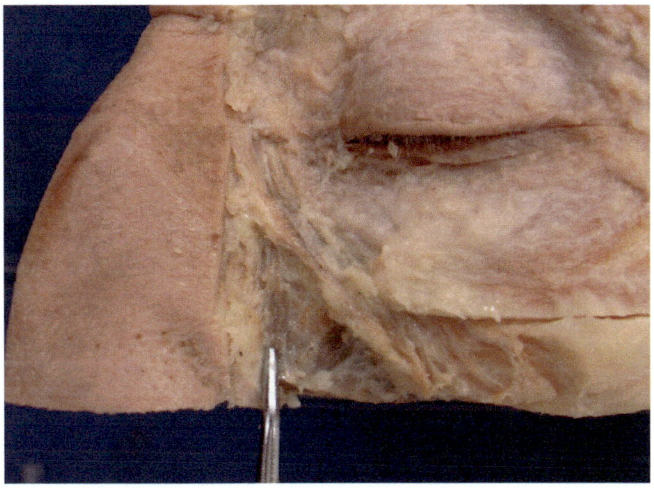

Fig. 2.19 Levator alae nasae muscle at pointer

8. Identify the orbital, preseptal, and pretarsal portions of the orbicularis oculi muscle of the upper eyelid (Figs. 2.20, 2.21, and 2.22) and of the lower eyelid (Figs. 2.23, 2.24, and 2.25).

Clinical correlation: Aggressive removal of the orbital and preseptal orbicularis is one treatment for essential blepharospasm. Injecting Botox is another treatment option.

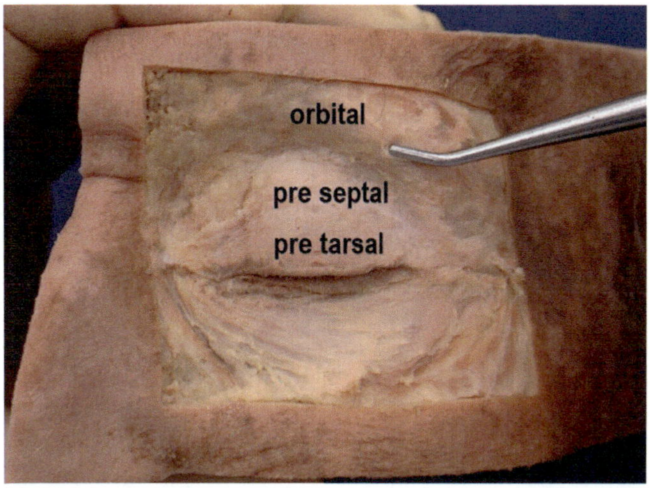

Fig. 2.20 The three arbitrary divisions of the orbicularis oculi muscle

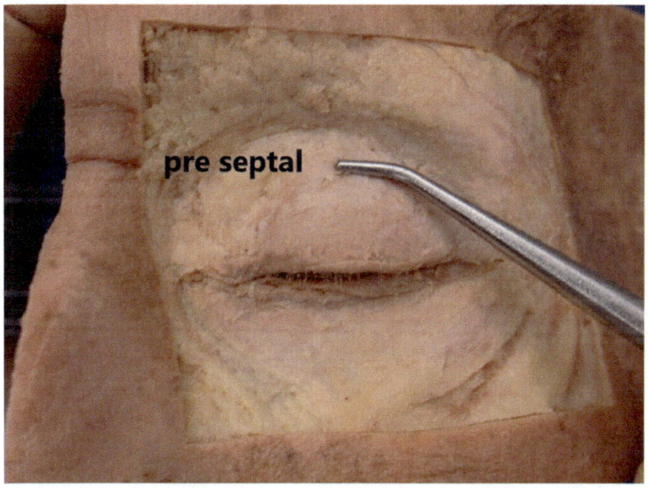

Fig. 2.21 The preseptal orbicularis oculi muscle of the upper lid

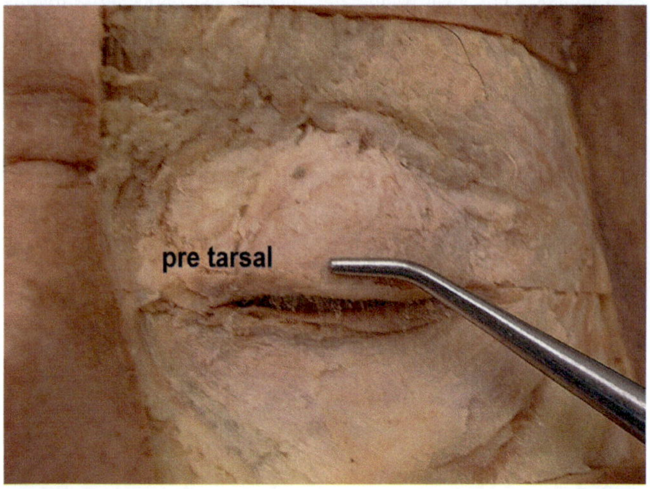

Fig. 2.22 The pretarsal orbicularis oculi muscle of the upper lid

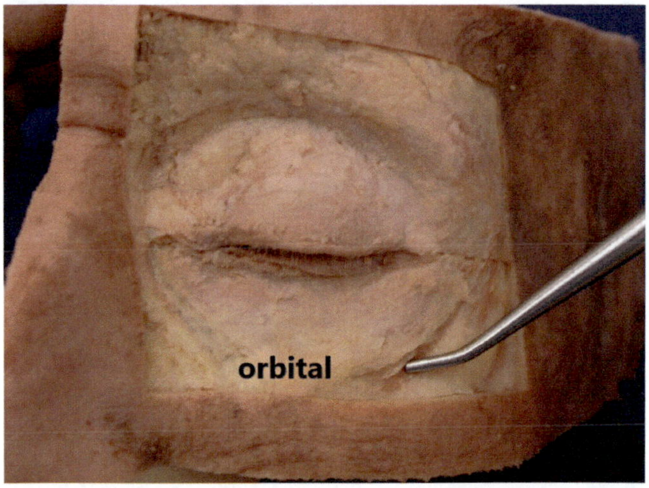

Fig. 2.23 The orbital orbicularis oculi muscle of the lower lid

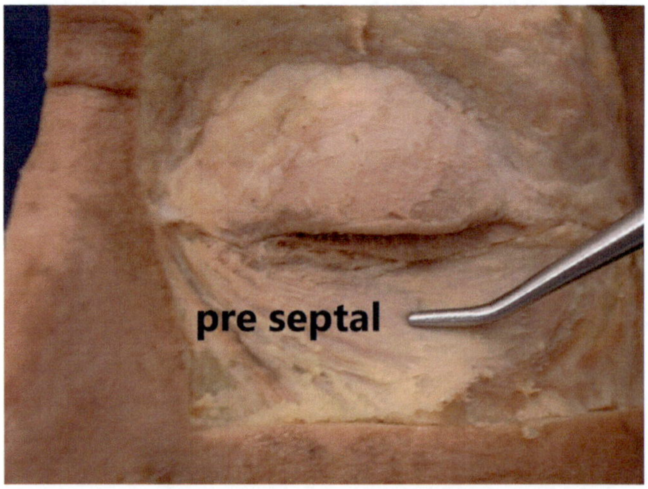

Fig. 2.24 The preseptal orbicularis oculi muscle of the lower lid

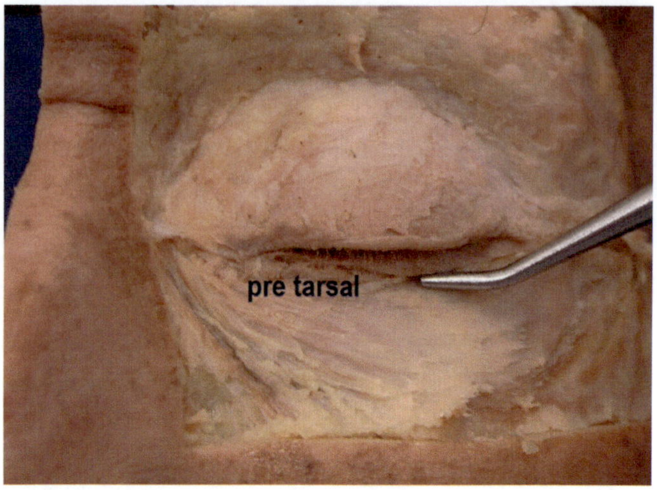

Fig. 2.25 The pretarsal orbicularis oculi muscle of the lower lid

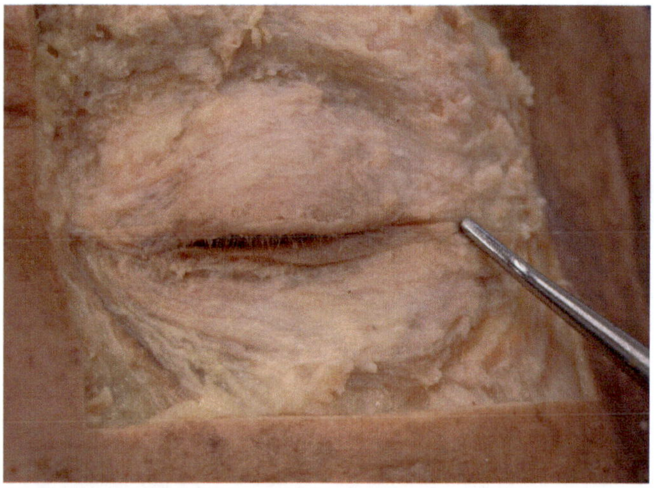

Fig. 2.26 The lateral palpebral raphe (pointer)

9. Note the lateral palpebral raphe (Fig. 2.26). This is where the orbicularis oculi muscle fibers of the upper and lower eyelids meet at the lateral canthal region.
10. Carefully identify and dissect the superficial temporal artery (Figs. 2.27, 2.28, and 2.29). Note its position deep to the skin and subcutaneous tissue, often in the superficial plane of the temporalis fascia, but superficial to the temporalis muscle.

Clinical correlation: Knowledge of the precise tissue plane of the superficial temporal artery is necessary when performing a temporal artery biopsy.

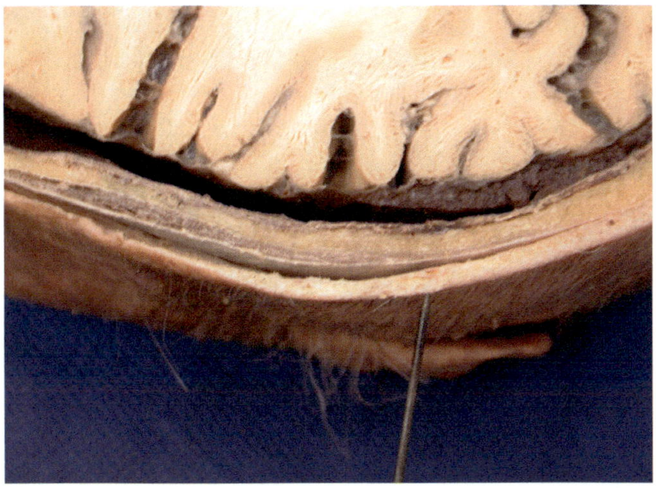

Fig. 2.27 Superficial temporal artery, deep to the skin, at end of pointer

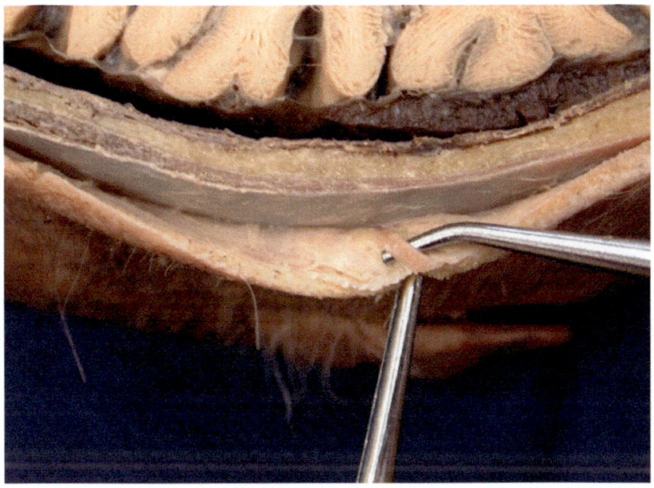

Fig. 2.28 Superficial temporal artery, deep to the skin and subcutaneous tissue

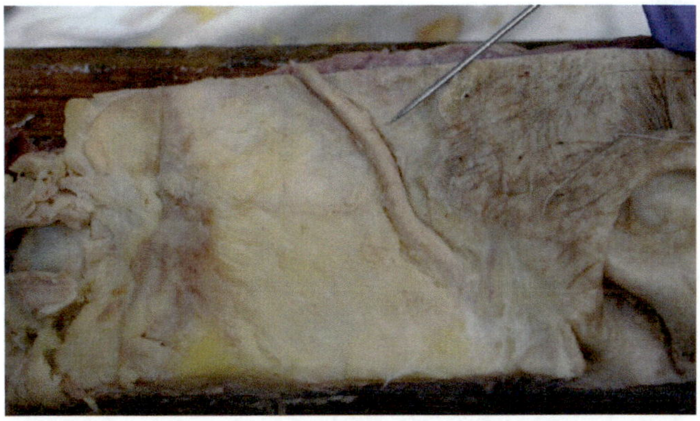

Fig. 2.29 Large superficial temporal artery, superficial to temporalis fascia

11. Dissect and identify the angular artery and vein (Fig. 2.30) inferior to the medial canthal tendon, between the levator alae nasae and levator labii superioris muscles.

Clinical correlation: Knowing the course of the angular vessels will help to control bleeding when operating in this region during external Dacyrocytorhinostomy (DCR), lower lid reconstruction, and medial canthal surgery.

12. Using a blade, make incisions into the muscle plane, outlining the frontalis and orbicularis oculi muscles, as with the skin incisions (Figs. 2.1 and 2.31).

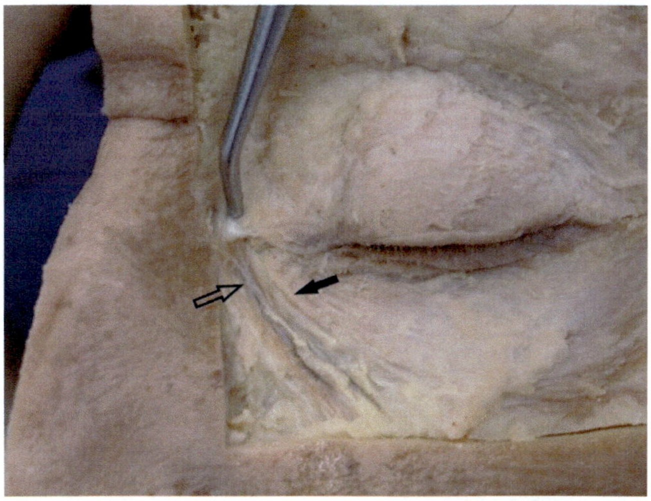

Fig. 2.30 Angular artery (solid arrow) and vein (hollow arrow). The pointer is on the medial canthal tendon

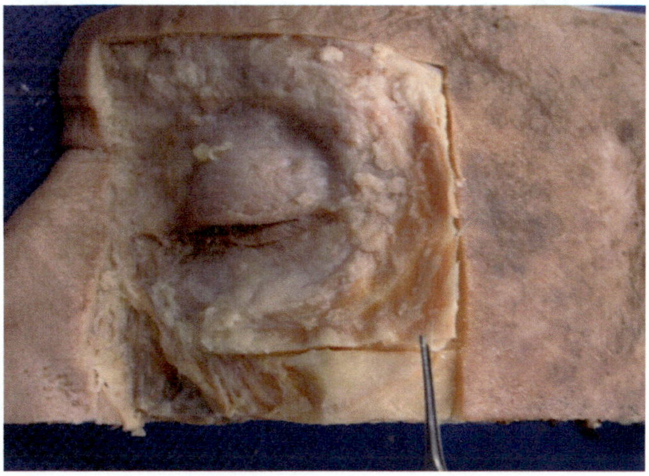

Fig. 2.31 Medial, temporal, superior, and inferior incisions through the orbital orbicularis muscle plane

13. Next dissect the muscle plane medially (Figs. 2.32 and 2.33), and reflect it toward the lid margin of the upper lid (Figs. 2.34 and 2.35) and the lower lid (Fig. 2.36). Care is needed to avoid dissecting too superficially and severing this thin muscle plane and also to avoid dissecting too deeply into posterior structures, i.e., orbital septum.

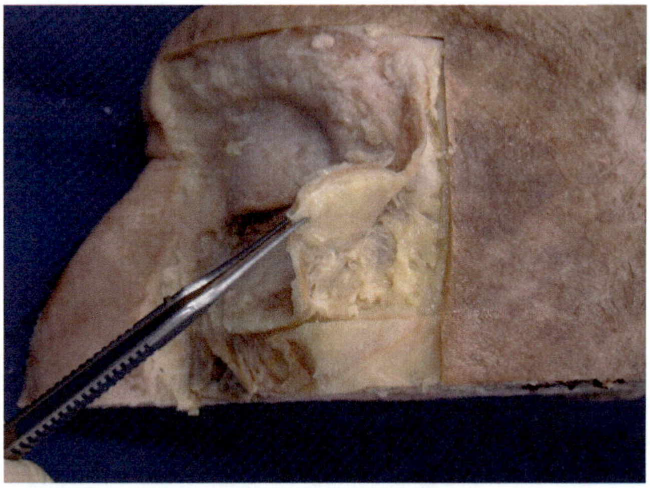

Fig. 2.32 Suborbicularis dissection starting temporally

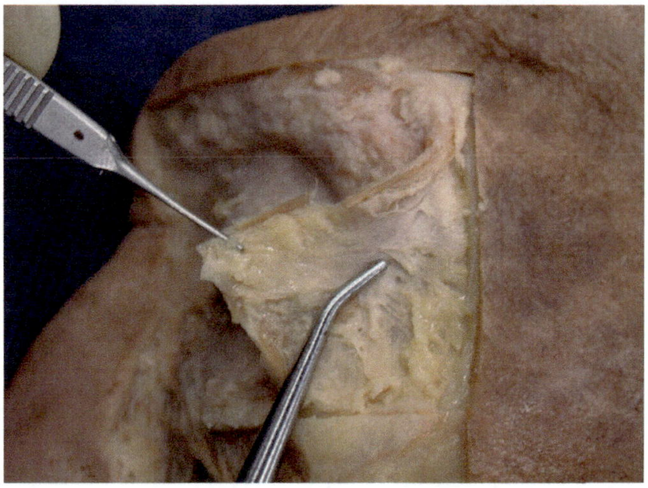

Fig. 2.33 Suborbicularis attachments (pointer) blending with the anterior horn of the lateral canthal tendon

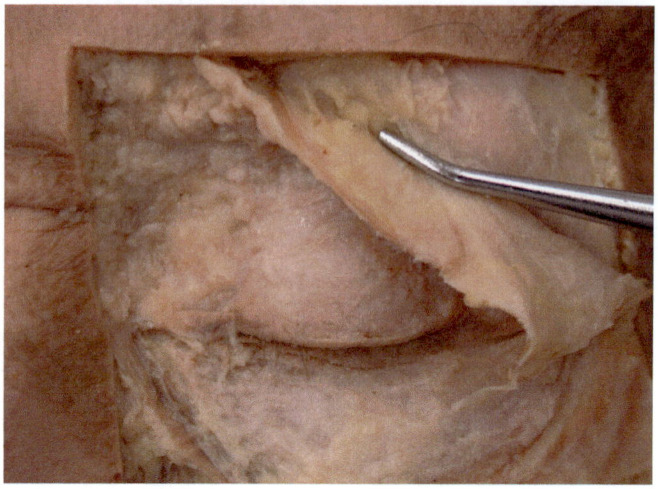

Fig. 2.34 Suborbicularis muscle plane dissected medially and toward the upper lid margin. Pointer is on the retro-orbicularis oculi fat (ROOF)

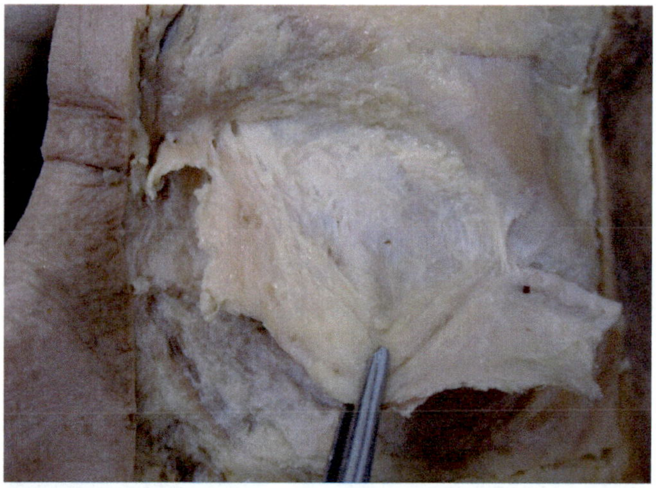

Fig. 2.35 Suborbicularis muscle plane dissected toward the upper lid margin

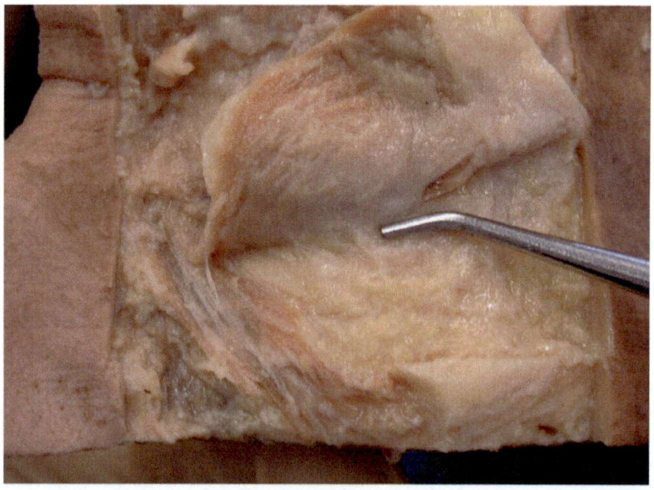

Fig. 2.36 Suborbicularis muscle plane dissected toward the lower lid margin. Pointer is on suborbicularis fascial attachments to orbital septum of the lower lid

14. Note the superficial fibrous extensions of the levator aponeurosis as they create the upper lid crease (Fig. 2.37) and the fibrous extensions of the lower lid retractors at the level of the lower lid crease. These fibrous insertions must be cut.

Clinical correlation: Surgically, if deep eyelid creases are desired, these fibrous attachments are recreated with deep supratarsal sutures during upper lid blepharoplasty or ptosis repair.

15. Identify the posterior lacrimal crest insertion of the pretarsal orbicularis (Fig. 2.38). These deep pretarsal orbicularis fibers are termed "Horner's muscle." Also note the deep preseptal fibers of the orbicularis, termed "Jones' muscle."

Clinical correlation: It is these deep pretarsal and preseptal orbicularis fibers that must be repositioned onto the posterior lacrimal crest at the time of trans-nasal wiring or medial canthal reconstruction to maintain the normal "concavity" at the medial canthus.

16. Expose the eyebrow fat pad, also named the retro-orbicularis oculi fat or "ROOF" (Fig. 2.39). It may, as in this specimen, descend into the eyelid, anterior to the septum.

Clinical correlation: Descended nasal brow fat pad is continuous with the posterior orbicularis fascia, anterior to the orbital septum. It can be mistaken for nasal *orbital* fat during blepharoplasty or external ptosis surgery.

17. Clean the superficial surface of superior and inferior orbital septa. Avoid going too deep.
18. Identify the supraorbital nerve in the region of the supraorbital notch (Fig. 2.40).

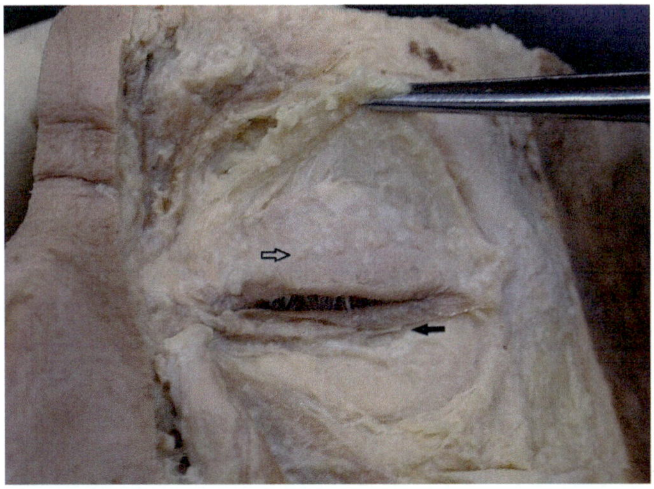

Fig. 2.37 With the orbicularis muscle plane reflected in the forceps, the cut superficial fibrous extensions of the levator aponeurosis (hollow arrow) and the superficial fibrous extensions of the lower lid retractors (solid arrow) are seen

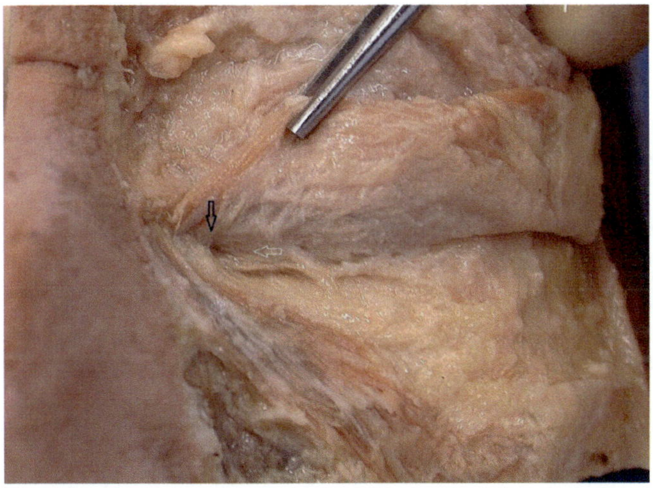

Fig. 2.38 Deep head of the pretarsal orbicularis muscle, Horner's muscle (white arrow). Deep head of the preseptal orbicularis muscle, Jones' muscle (black arrow)

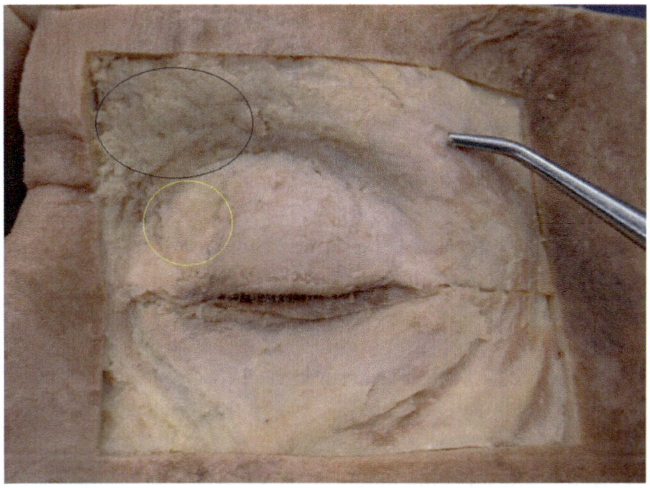

Fig. 2.39 With the orbicularis muscle plane removed, the retro-orbicularis oculi fat (ROOF) (black circle) extends into the lid (yellow) anterior to the septum. The pointer is on the superior orbital rim

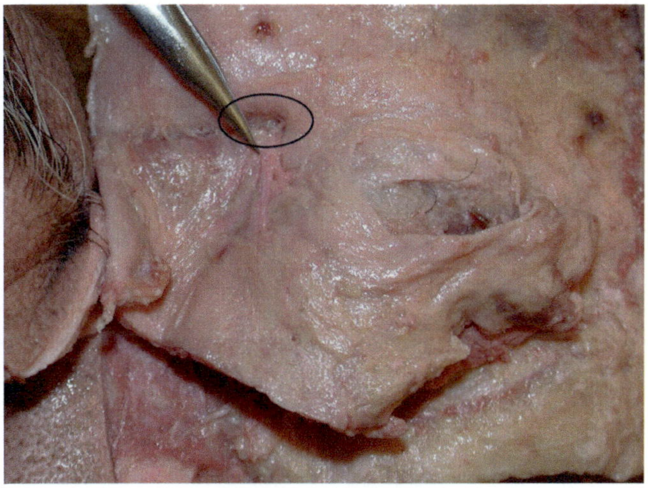

Fig. 2.40 Supraorbital nerve (pointer) exiting from the supraorbital notch (circle)

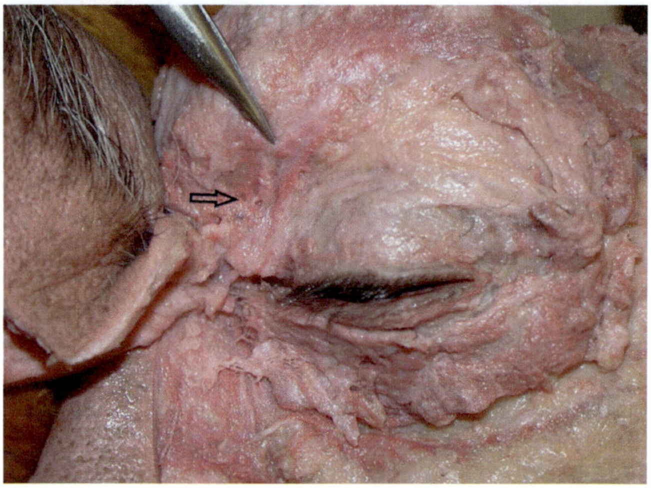

Fig. 2.41 Supratrochlear nerve (arrow) and artery as they pierce the corrugator supercilii (pointer)

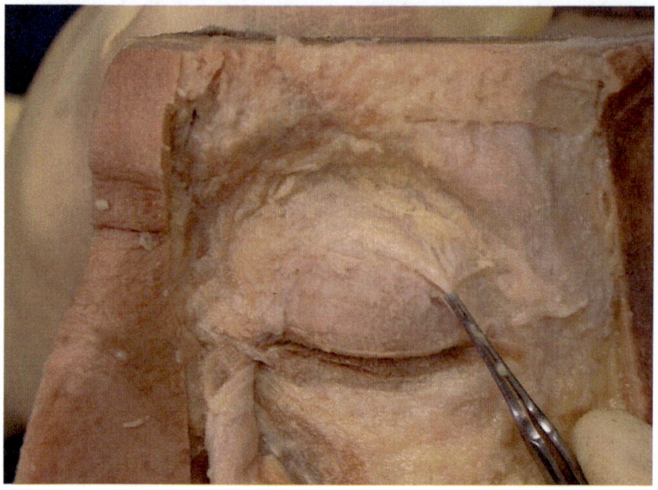

Fig. 2.42 Orbital septum of the upper eyelid in forceps, tented anteriorly

19. Identify the supratrochlear nerve and artery Eyelidssupretrochlear nerve and artery as they pierce the corrugator supercilii (Fig. 2.41).
20. Identify the infratrochlear nerve below the trochlea. It may be difficult to identify.

Clinical correlations:

(a) Sites for supraorbital, supratrochlear, and infratrochlear nerve blocks for local anesthesia.
(b) These nerves are to be protected during brow lift surgery to prevent post-op hypesthesia.
(c) Nerve distribution of herpes zoster ophthalmicus.

Clinical Correlation: knowledge of this anatomy is important when performing neurotonization of the supraorbital nerve for neurotrophic keratitis

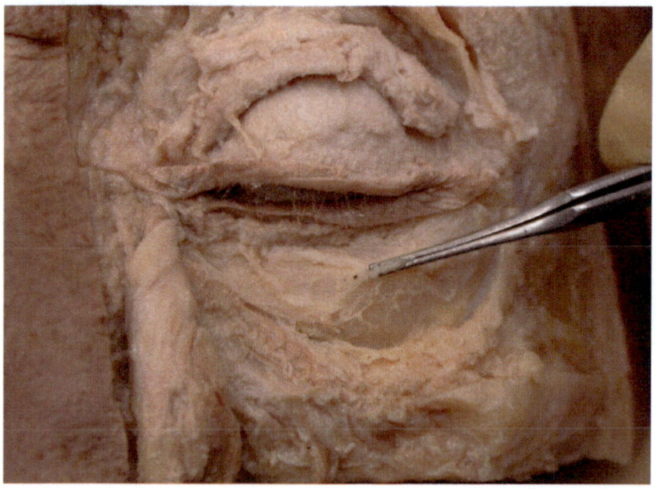

Fig. 2.43 Orbital septum of the lower eyelid in forceps, tented anteriorly

Upper Lid Septum and Levator Aponeurosis

21. Identify the septum of the upper lid (Fig. 2.42) and of the lower lid (Fig. 2.43) by "tenting" the tissue anteriorly.
22. The dense fibrous condensation where the periorbita within the orbit meets the periosteum of the frontal bone at the orbital rim is termed the *arcus marginalis*. The orbital septum is an extension of this confluence into the eyelid. Leaving the palpebral attachments of the orbital septum intact, incise the superior orbital septum at the arcus marginalis at the superior orbital rim (Figs. 2.44 and 2.45).

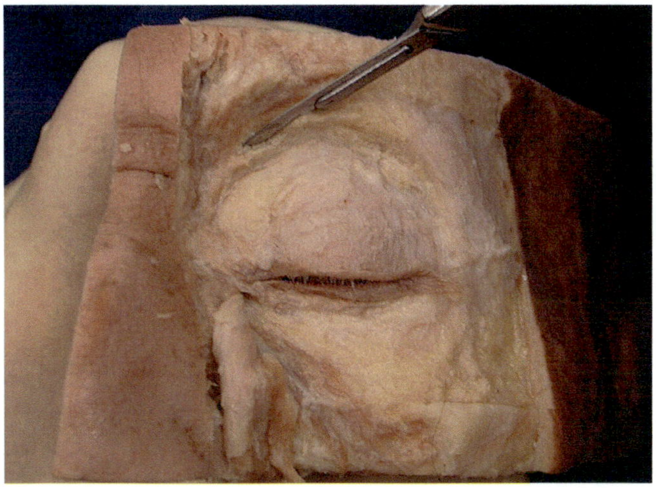

Fig. 2.44 Periosteal incision at arcus marginalis of nasal superior orbital rim

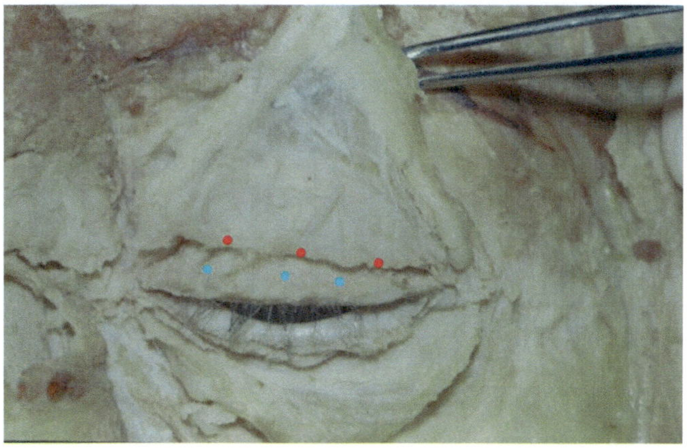

Fig. 2.46 The thin orbital septum of the upper lid (anterior to the forceps) is dissected at the arcus marginalis but remains attached to the anterior surface of the levator aponeurosis (red dots), already dissected from the tarsus (blue dots)

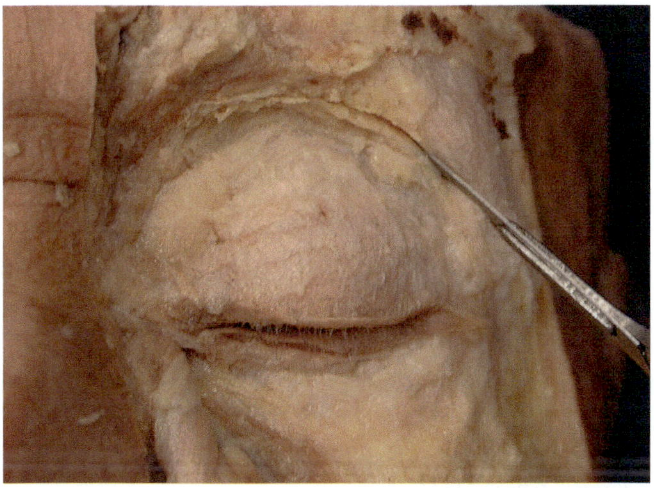

Fig. 2.45 Periosteal incision at arcus marginalis of temporal superior orbital rim

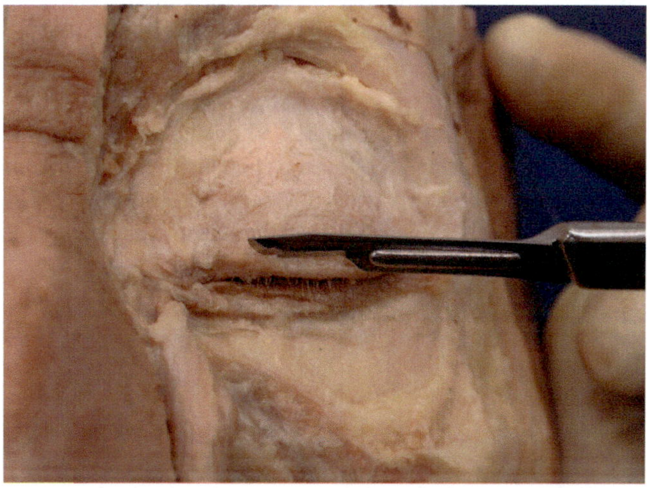

Fig. 2.47 Medial incision through levator attachments to tarsus

23. Beginning superiorly and with scissors posterior to the septum of the upper lid, carefully elevate the thin septum inferiorly toward the lid margin (Fig. 2.46).
24. Note how the orbital septum inserts or attaches to the anterior surface of the levator aponeurosis, and not to the superior tarsus.
25. Make an incision 2 mm above the superior eyelid margin, medially to laterally, through the levator aponeurosis insertion onto the anterior surface of the tarsus (Figs. 2.47 and 2.48).

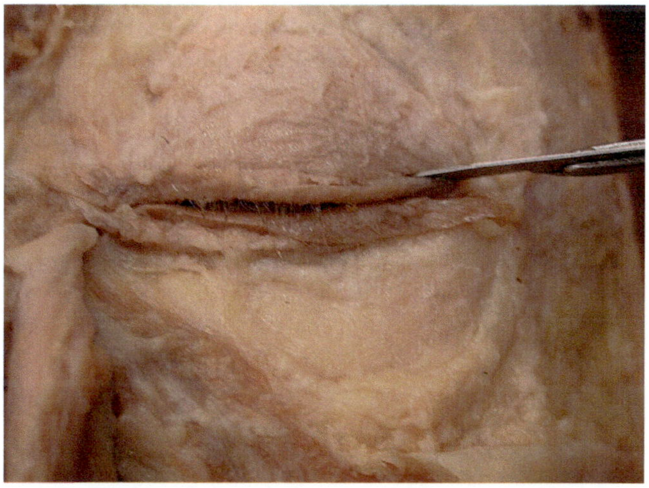

Fig. 2.48 Lateral incision through levator attachments to tarsus

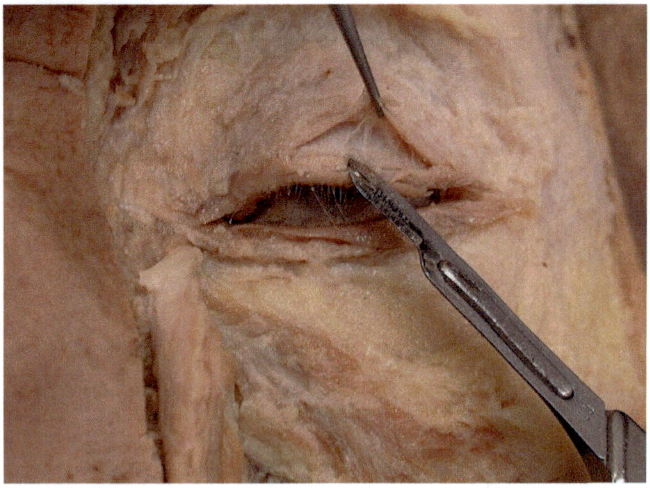

Fig. 2.49 Dissection of levator aponeurosis from the anterior surface of the tarsus

26. Beginning at the lid margin, superiorly dissect the levator aponeurosis from the anterior tarsal surface (Fig. 2.49).

Clinical correlation: Understanding the relationship of the orbital septum and the levator aponeurosis will enhance the results of blepharoplasty and external ptosis surgery. The orbital septum is penetrated to gain surgical access to the superior orbital fat and levator aponeurosis.

Tarsus

27. Note the height (10 mm) and width of the superior tarsus.

Clinical correlation: Free tarsal grafts can be harvested as a spacer in the correction of lid retraction or for lid reconstruction.

28. Identify the marginal arterial arcade on the anterior surface of the tarsus, approximately 3 mm from the lid margin (Fig. 2.50).

Clinical correlation: Knowing the location of this artery during lid margin surgery or traumatic lid laceration repair will allow the surgeon to control intraoperative bleeding and allow a dry operative field. Eyelid margin vascularity is presevered during tarsal graft harvesting by leaving intact a 4mm marginal tarsal segment containing the artery.

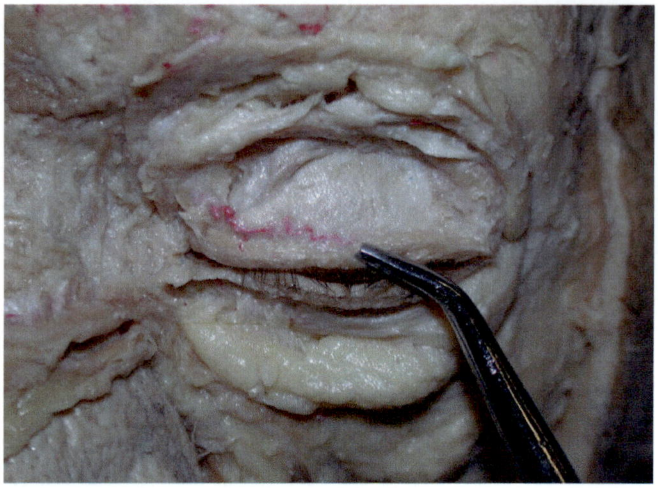

Fig. 2.50 Marginal artery of the upper lid

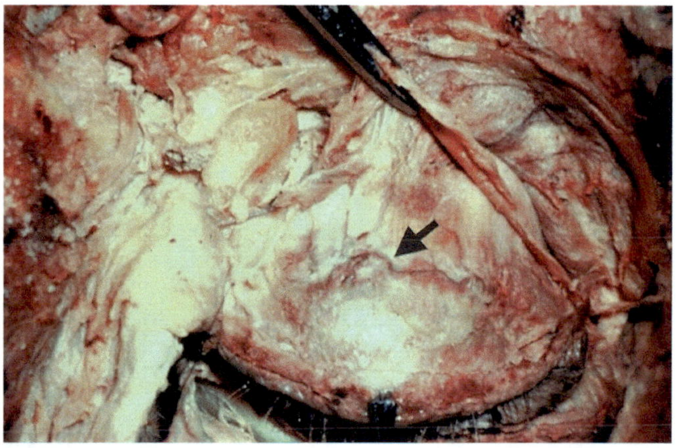

Fig. 2.51 Peripheral artery of the upper lid (arrow). The levator aponeurosis is reflected in forceps

29. Identify the "peripheral arterial arcade" superior to the tarsus, but posterior to the levator aponeurosis (Fig. 2.51) and anterior to Müller's muscle.

Clinical correlation: Knowing the location of this artery during ptosis surgery or retractor repair surgery will allow for a less bloody operative field.

Müller's Muscle

30. With inferior traction of the upper eyelid, continue superior pretarsal dissection in a plane posterior to the levator aponeurosis (Fig. 2.52). Loose attachments from the posterior surface of the levator will be lysed, so as to separate the levator from the underlying superior tarsal muscle of Müller.
31. Identify Müller's muscle insertion on the superior edge of the tarsus (Fig. 2.53) .This sympathetically innervated muscle originates from the posterior surface of the levator approximately 12 mm above the tarsus (Fig. 2.54).

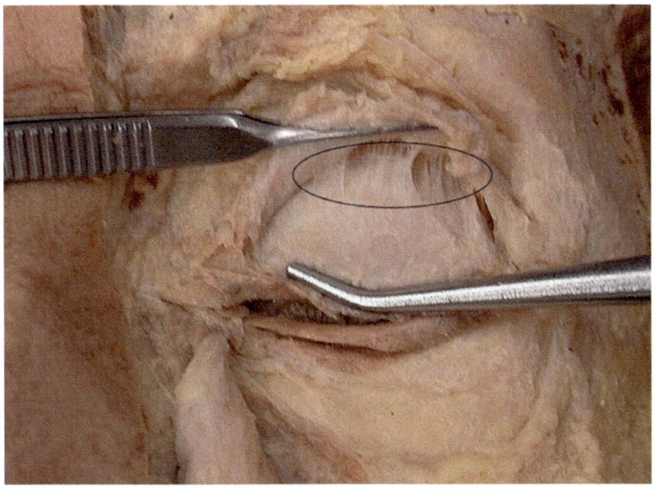

Fig. 2.52 Loose attachments (circle) from the posterior surface of the levator aponeurosis (in forceps to the anterior surface of Müller's muscle)

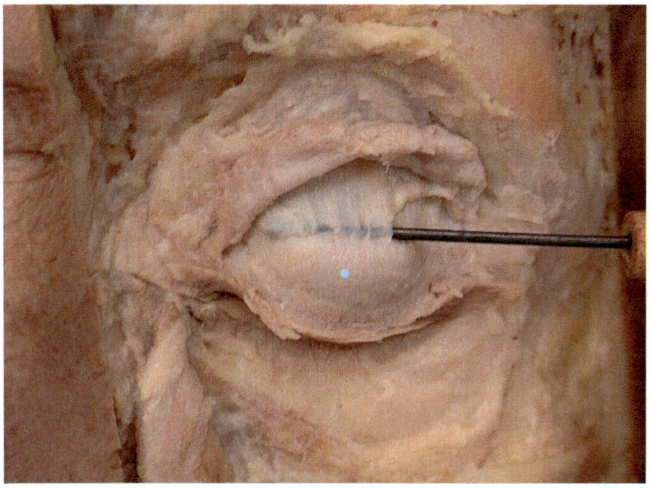

Fig. 2.53 Müller's muscle, anterior to the pointer, inserting onto the superior edge of the tarsus (blue dot)

Fig. 2.54 Cross-sectional drawing of the upper eyelid. Müller's muscle is drawn in purple, the tarsus is in blue, and the suspensory ligament to the superior fornix is in dark green

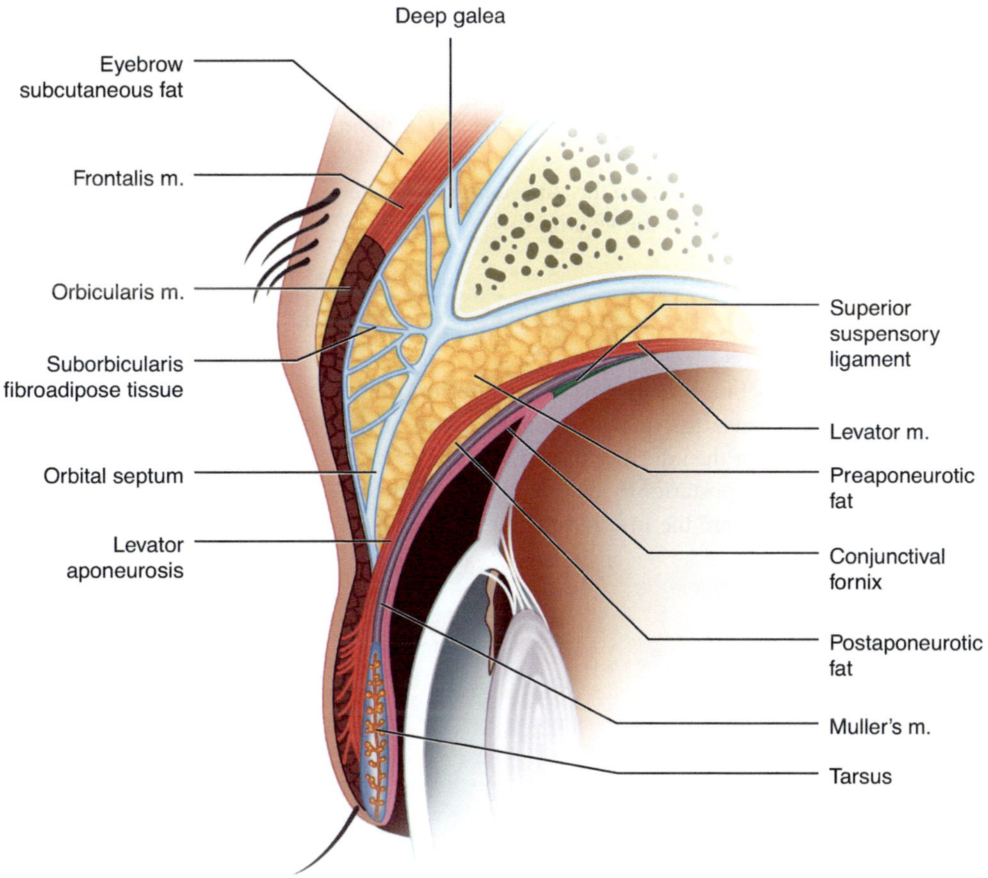

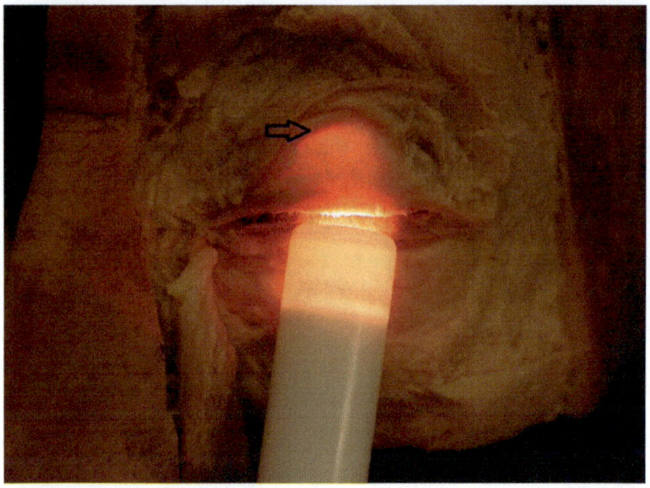

Fig. 2.55 Retroillumination of superior fornix (arrow)

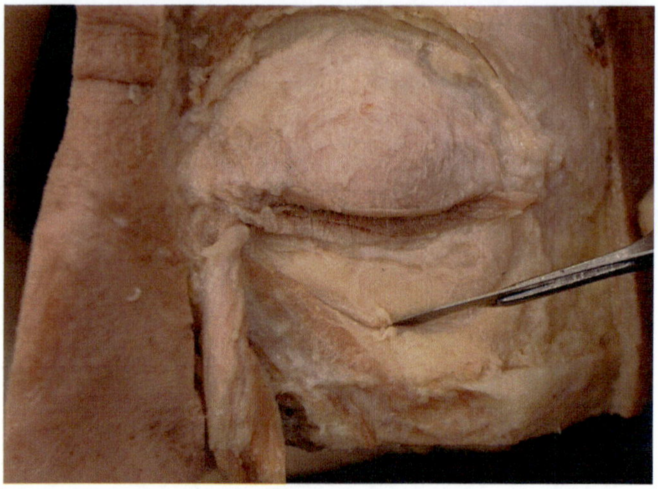

Fig. 2.56 Incision at inferior orbital rim through arcus marginalis

Clinical correlation:

(a) A procedure to correct 1–2 mm of blepharoptosis is to shorten Müller's muscle, thus elevating the eyelid.
(b) A procedure to correct eyelid retraction is to detach Müller's muscle from its insertion at the superior edge of the tarsus, thus lowering the eyelid.

32. Note the suspensory ligament of the superior fornix (Fig. 2.54), just superior to the origin of Müller's muscle, attaching the conjunctival fornix to the underside of the levator.
33. Place a smooth flat instrument into the superior conjunctival fornix to identify its position. The same can be done by retro-illumination (Fig. 2.55).
34. Remove Müller's muscle from the superior tarsal border and from the underside of the levator.

Lower Lid Septum

35. Leaving the palpebral attachments of the inferior orbital septum intact, incise the inferior orbital septum at the arcus marginalis of the inferior orbital rim (Fig. 2.56).
36. Then with scissors posterior to the septum, carefully dissect superiorly toward the inferior edge of the tarsus of the lower lid (Fig. 2.57). Before reaching the inferior tarsal border, the septum fuses with the lower lid retractors as the conjoint tendon. The conjoint tendon then attaches to the lower edge of the lower tarsus.

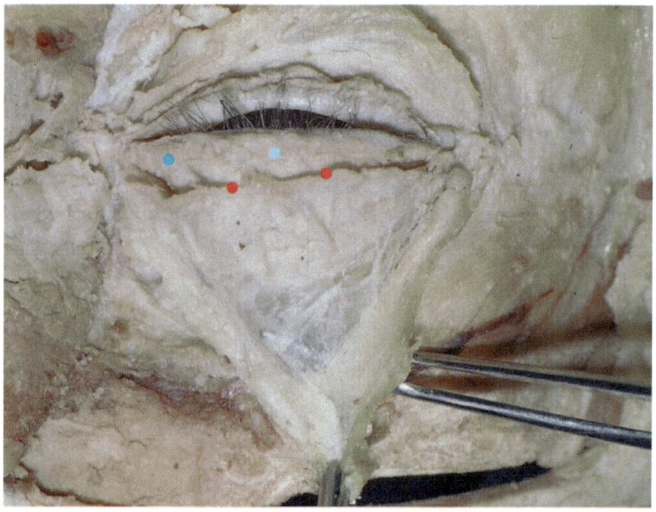

Fig. 2.57 The forceps are seen through a very thin inferior orbital septum, dissected free at the inferior arcus marginalis. The septum is still attached to the conjoint tendon, the confluence of the septum and lower lid retractors (red dots), near the lower border of the tarsus (blue dots)

Lower Lid Retractors and Tarsus

37. Note that the height of the inferior tarsus (5 mm) is half that of the superior tarsus (10 mm).
38. Identify the lower lid retractors at the inferior border of the lower lid tarsus (Figs. 2.58 and 2.59). Depressing the anteriorly located orbital fat of the lower lid may help. Collectively, the capsulopalpebral fascia and the inferior tarsus muscle are known as the lower lid retractors.

Clinical correlation:

(a) Reattachment of dehisced lower lid retractors to the lower edge of the tarsus is the anatomically correct surgical procedure for "tarsal ectropion."
(b) Knowing the relationship of the lower tarsal border, the conjoint tendon, the lower lid retractors, and the orbital septum is helpful for the correction of lower lid retraction.

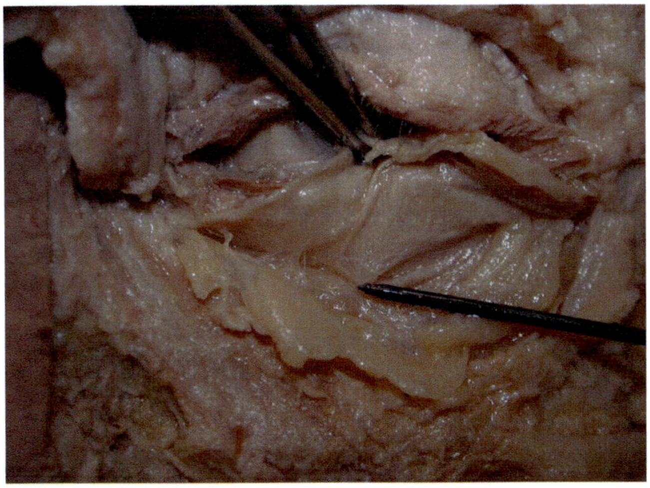

Fig. 2.58 Lower lid retractors (pointer). The inferior orbital septum is reflected superiorly in the forceps

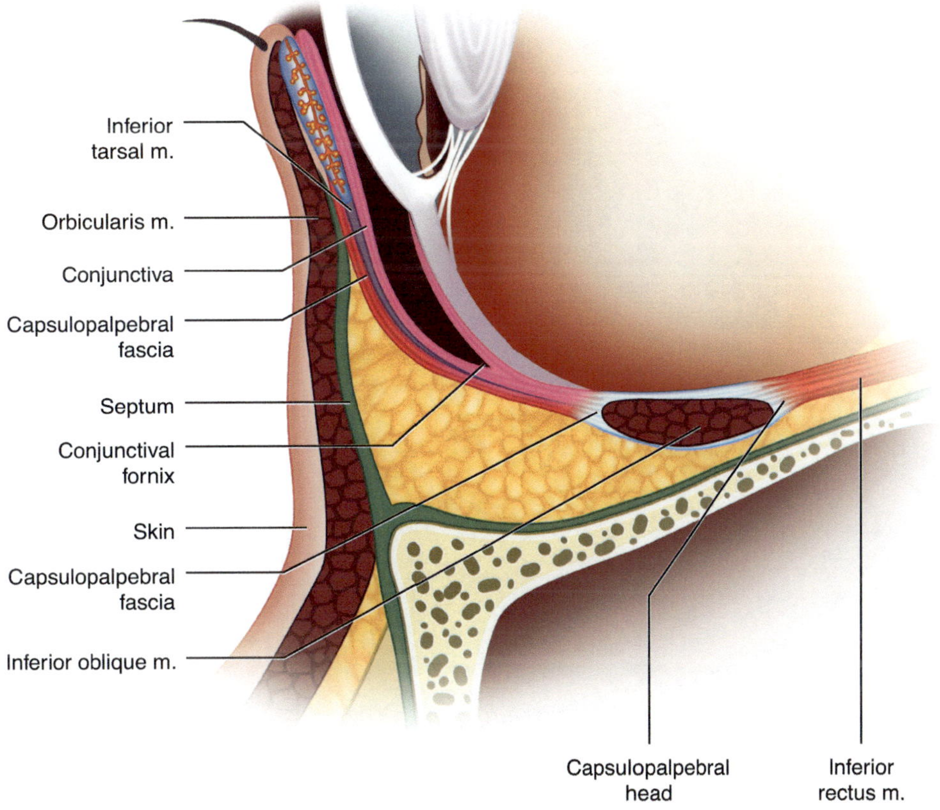

Fig. 2.59 Cross-sectional drawing of the lower eyelid. Collectively, the capsulopalpebral fascia, drawn in red, and the inferior tarsus muscle, drawn in purple, are known as the lower lid retractors. About 5 mm below the lower tarsal border, the lower lid retractors fuse with the septum (green) as the conjoint tendon and together attach to the lower border of the tarsus

Lateral Canthal Tendon

39. Identify the lateral canthal tendon (Fig. 2.60) inserting approximately 4 mm inside the lateral orbital rim at the tubercle of Whitnall. Occasionally, a small pocket of fat "Isler's fat pocket" is found posterior to the anterior horn of the lateral canthal tendon.

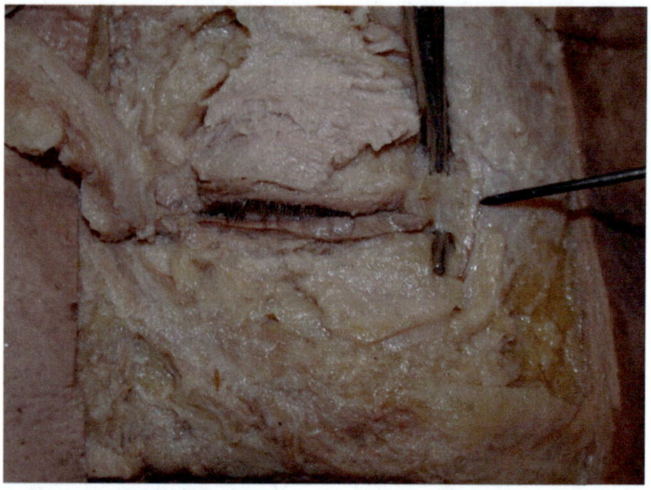

Fig. 2.60 The anterior horn of the lateral canthal tendon is seen anterior to the probe. The pointer is on the lateral orbital rim

Clinical correlation: A surgically created "lateral tarsal strip" must be reattached inside the lateral orbital rim at the tubercle of Whitnall to maintain normal lateral canthal contour to maintain normal lateral eyelid contact with the eye. A lateral tarsal strip is often used for the correction of ectropion, lower lid laxity, lateral canthal tendon laxity, and occasionally entropion.

Suggested Reading

Anderson RL, Gordy DD. The tarsal strip procedure. Arch Ophthalmol. 1979;97(11):2192–6.

Beard C, Quickert M. Anatomy of the orbit. second ed. Birmingham, AL: Aesculapius Publishing Company; 1977. p. 2–14.

Bedrossian EH Jr. Embryology and anatomy of the eyelid. In: Tasman W, Jaeger E, editors. Foundations of clinical ophthalmology, vol. 1. Philadelphia: Lippincott; 1998. p. 1–23.

Della Rocca RC, Bedrossian EH, Arthurs BP. Ophthalmic plastic surgery: decision making and techniques. New York: McGraw Hill; 2002. p. 25–40.

Whitnall SE. The levator palpebrae superioris muscle: the attachments and relations of its aponeurosis. Ophthalmoscope. 1914;12:258–63.

Anterior Orbit

3

Edward H. Bedrossian, Jr

The orbital septum separates the eyelid from the orbit. In this chapter, dissection of the eyelids will continue in more detail posterior to the septum into the anterior orbit. The fat pads will be identified, and the levator aponeurosis and lower lid retractors will be further dissected. Clinical correlation will be provided.

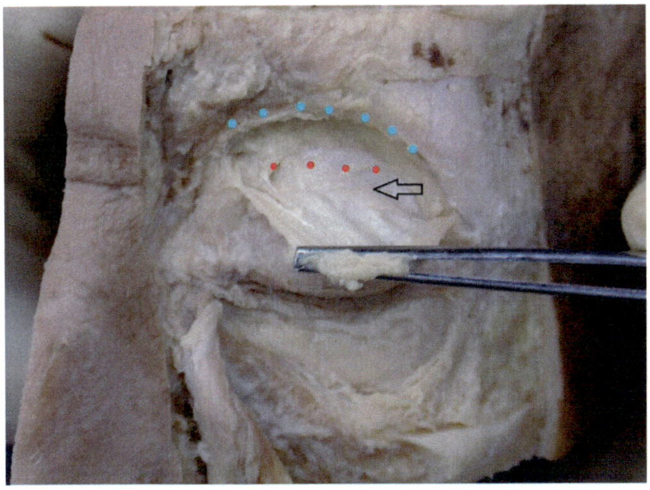

Fig. 3.1 Inferiorly reflected orbital septum (in forceps) dissected from arcus marginalis (blue dots) attached (arrow) to the anterior surface of the levator aponeurosis (red dots)

Orbital Septum of the Upper Lid

1. With the superior orbital septum (Fig. 3.1) dissected from the arcus marginalis at the superior orbital rim and reflected inferiorly, note the attachment of the superior orbital septum with the levator aponeurosis.

With the septum retracted superiorly (Fig. 3.2), note that its insertion to the levator aponeurosis "prevents" the septum from reaching the superior tarsal border.

Clinical correlation: The orbital septum of the upper lid is left open during upper lid blepharoplasty surgery, ptosis repair, and upper lid reconstruction to avoid postoperative upper lid retraction.

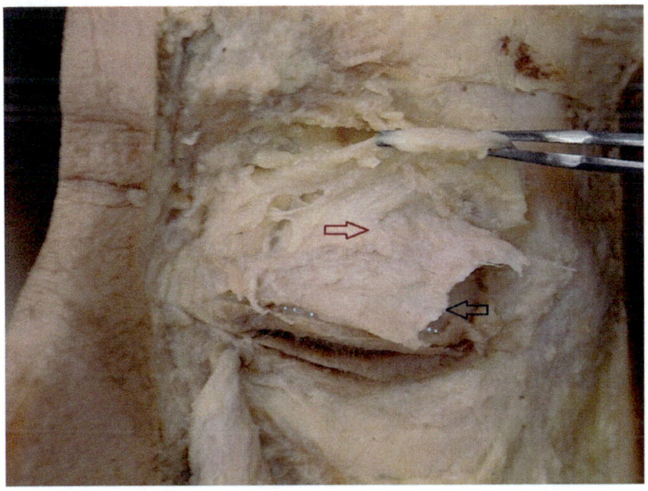

Fig. 3.2 Superiorly retracted orbital septum (in forceps) with attachments (red arrow) to anterior surface of the levator aponeurosis (black arrow), detached from tarsus (blue dots)

E. H. Bedrossian, Jr, MD, FACS (✉)
Wills Eye Hospital, Philadelphia, PA, USA

E. H. Bedrossian, Jr et al. (eds.), *Anatomy of the Eyelid, Orbit, and Lacrimal System*,
https://doi.org/10.1007/978-3-030-88265-5_3

Fat Pads of the Upper Lid

2. Immediately beneath the superior orbital septum lies a fat layer (Fig. 3.3) consisting of a smaller fibrous medial (nasal) pad and a larger more lobular and central (pre-aponeurotic) fat pad, separated by the trochlea. The trochlea can be first identified by palpation and then by blunt dissection of the fat.
3. Dissect the fat pads (Fig. 3.4). Note the medial fat pad and the central/pre-aponeurotic fat pad.
4. Identify the trochlea (Fig. 3.5). Dissect and identify the reflected superior oblique tendon.

Clinical correlation:

(a) The pre-aponeurotic fat pad (Fig. 3.6) serves as an important landmark to the levator aponeurosis during surgery because it lies immediately above and anterior to the levator aponeurosis.
(b) The medial fat pad is highly vascular and has attachments to the posterior orbital fat. Meticulous hemostasis is needed during medial fat management during cosmetic blepharoplasty. The pre-aponeurotic fat pad is less vascular and does not attach to posterior orbital fat.

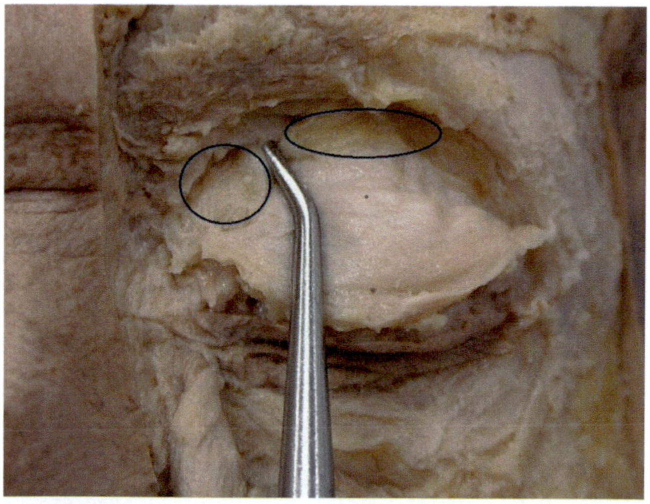

Fig. 3.3 Medial fat pad (circle) and central fat pad (oval). The pointer is on the trochlea

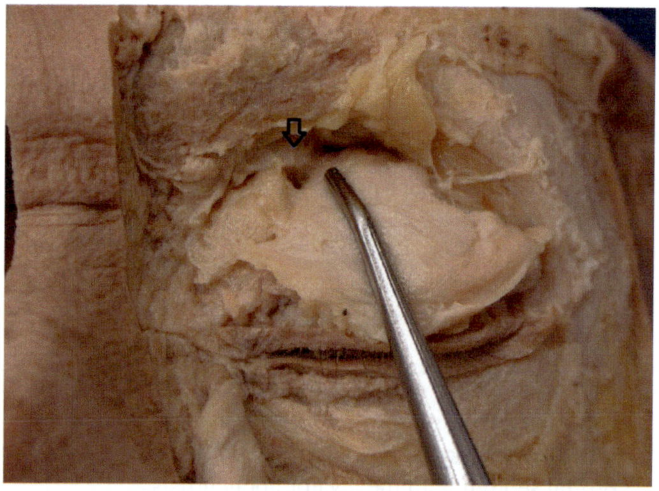

Fig. 3.5 Trochlea (arrow). Superior oblique tendon (pointer)

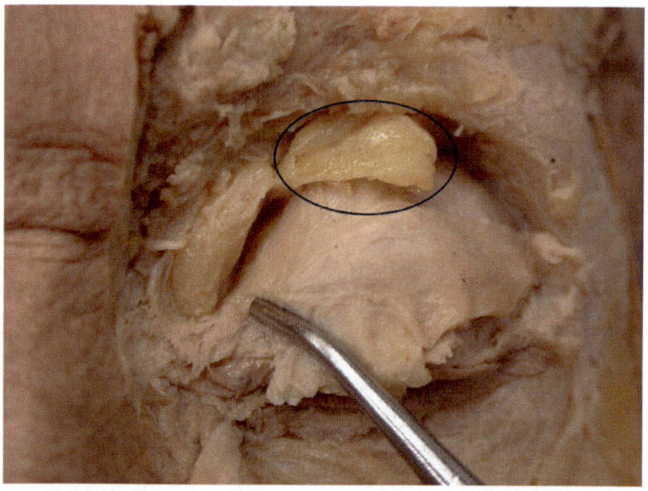

Fig. 3.4 Medial fat pad (pointer) and central fat pad (oval). The central fat pad is also called the pre-aponeurotic fat pad

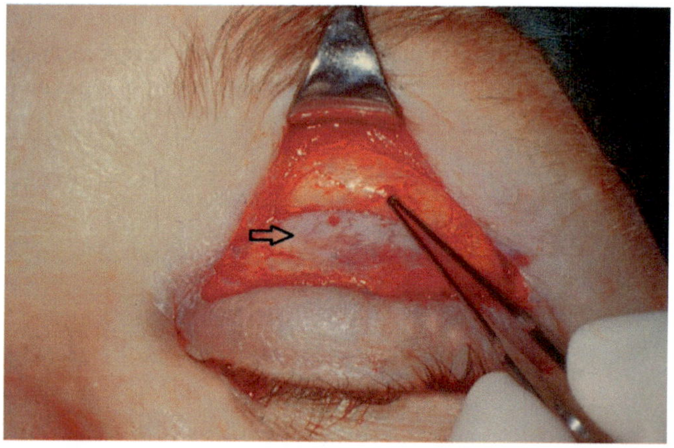

Fig. 3.6 Surgical slide. The yellow pre-aponeurotic fat pad (pointer) is seen anterior to the whiter levator aponeurosis (arrow)

Levator Aponeurosis

5. Examine the levator aponeurosis (Fig. 3.7). Note the lateral extension or "horn" of the levator aponeurosis dividing the lacrimal gland as the levator courses to the lateral orbital tubercle.
6. Palpate the lateral orbital tubercle (also called Whitnall's orbital tubercle) as a small protuberance 2–4 mm inside the lateral orbital rim.
7. Identify the smaller palpebral lobe (Fig. 3.8) and the larger orbital lobe (Fig. 3.9) of the lacrimal gland.

Clinical correlation: During fat management for blepharoplasty, it is important to note that the anterior portion of the orbital lobe of the lacrimal gland lies in the same plane as the medial and central fat pads (Fig. 3.9). It is not mistaken as orbital fat by its pink color and lateral location. Accidental removal may cause or aggravate dry eye syndrome.

8. Identify the medial horn of the levator (Fig. 3.10) joining the medial retinaculum to insert on the posterior lacrimal crest.

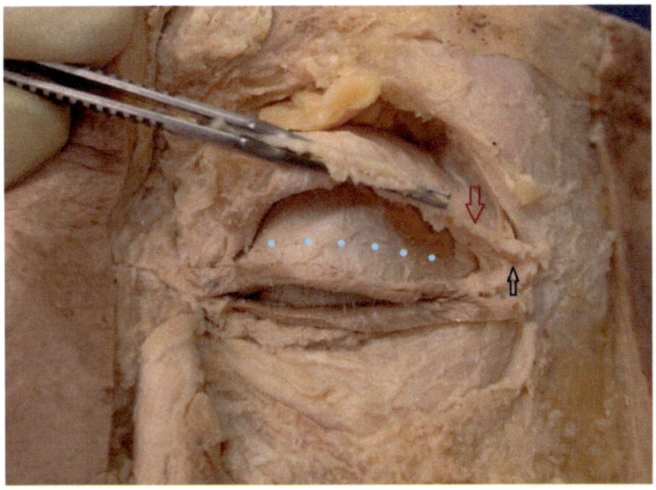

Fig. 3.7 Levator aponeurosis (in forceps) dissected from anterior surface of tarsus (blue dots). Lateral horn of the levator aponeurosis (red arrow) is attached to the lateral orbital tubercle (black arrow)

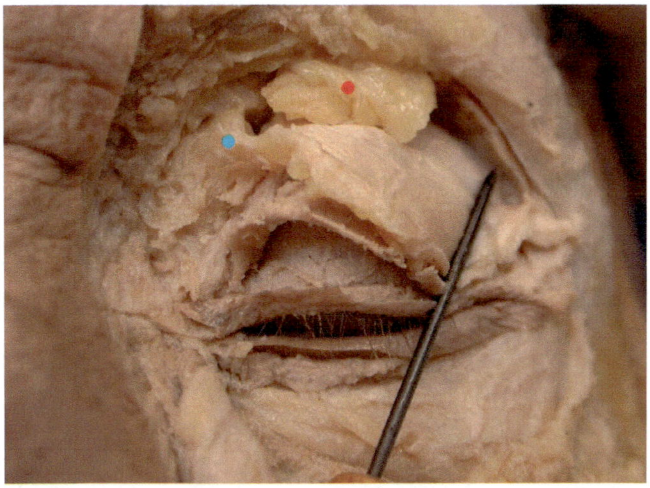

Fig. 3.9 Anterior edge of the orbital lobe of the lacrimal gland (pointer). Note the medial fat pad (blue dot) and central fat pad (red dot)

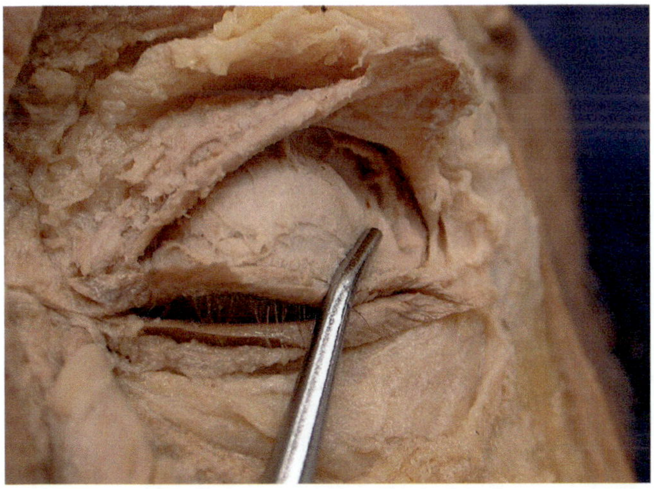

Fig. 3.8 Palpebral lobe of the lacrimal gland

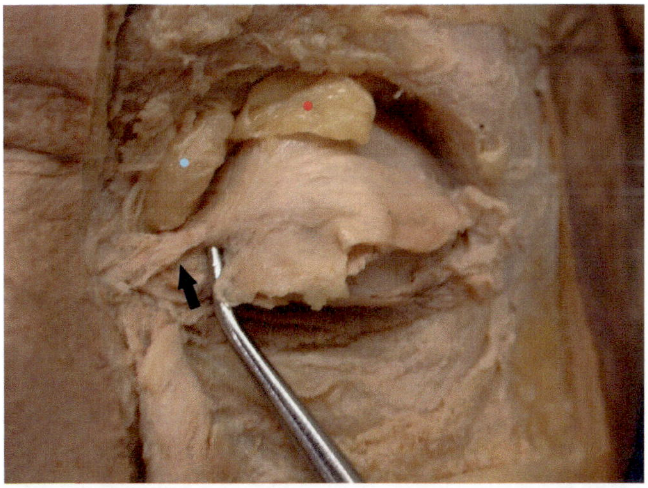

Fig. 3.10 Medial horn of levator (pointer), joining the medial retinaculum (arrow). Note the medial fat pad (blue dot) and central fat pad (red dot)

Clinical correlation: During levator surgery for the correction of blepharoptosis, the lateral and medial horns are usually left in place to enhance the effect of the ptosis correction.

9. Note the confluence of the superior orbital septum with the levator aponeurosis (Figs. 3.11 and 3.12).
10. Next, inferiorly reflect the septum and the attached levator aponeurosis. Then excise the medial and preaponeurotic fat pads.
11. Further superior dissection of the levator aponeurosis reveals a white band, the superior transverse ligament of Whitnall (Fig. 3.13), extending from its medial attachment at the trochlea to its primary lateral attachments at the frontozygomatic suture. Note its secondary attachments to Whitnall's orbital tubercle.

Orbital Septum of the Lower Lid

12. Reflect the inferior orbital septum (Fig. 3.14) superiorly to the conjoint tendon and its insertion at the inferior edge of the lower tarsus. The conjoint tendon represents the fusion of the septum with the lower lid retractors, 5 mm below the lower edge of the tarsus.

Clinical correlation: The orbital septum is left open when preforming orbital floor fracture repair, lower lid blepharoplasty and lid reconstruction, to avoid postoperative lower lid retraction.

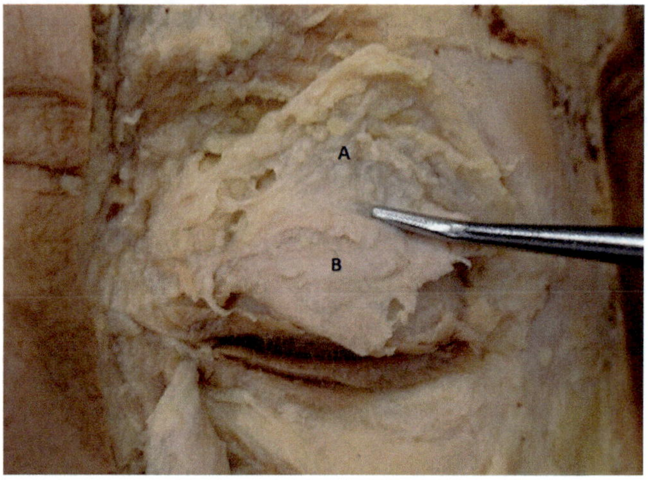

Fig. 3.11 Orbital septum (**a**) with attachments (pointer) to levator aponeurosis (**b**)

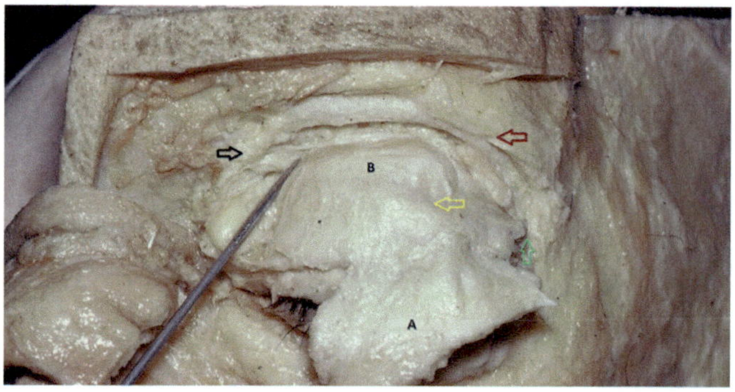

Fig. 3.13 Whitnall's ligament (white band above pointer) extending from the trochlea (black arrow) to the frontozygomatic suture (red arrow). Note its secondary attachments to Whitnall's orbital tubercle (green arrow). Also note the inferiorly reflected septum (**a**) with attachments (yellow arrow) to the levator aponeurosis (**b**)

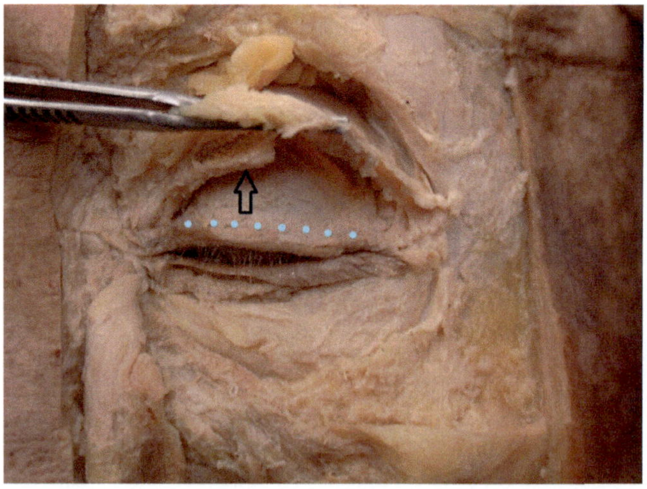

Fig. 3.12 Orbital septum (in forceps) attached to levator aponeurosis (arrow). The levator aponeurosis has been dissected from the tarsus (blue dots)

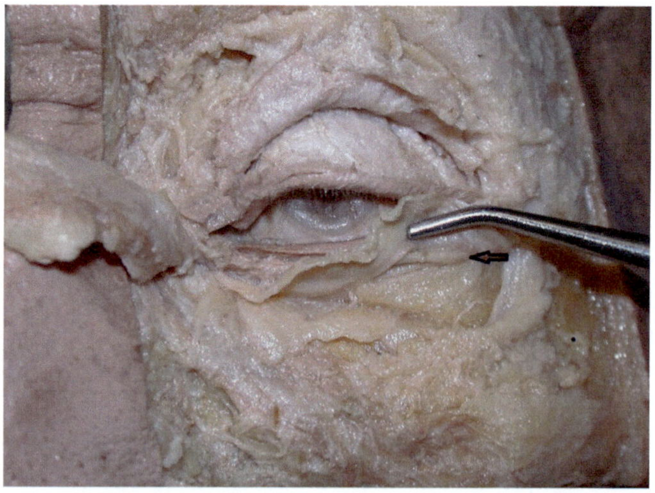

Fig. 3.14 Septum of lower lid, dissected from the arcus marginalis at inferior orbital rim and then reflected superiorly by pointer, exposing the inferior tarsal border (arrow)

Fat Pads of the Lower Lid

13. Posterior to the septum, note the exposed inferior orbital fat pads (Fig. 3.15).
14. Identify a larger medial and a smaller temporal (or lateral) fat pad (Fig. 3.15). The division between the two (Fig. 3.15) is formed by a fascial band extending from the periorbita and orbital septum infra-laterally, joining to the capsulopalpebral fascia and Lockwood's ligament supramedially.
15. The medial fat pad extends from this fascial band to the medial canthal area. The medial fat fad is a single pad anteriorly but is divided posteriorly into a nasal and a central fat pad by the inferior oblique muscle (Fig. 3.16). The inferior oblique muscle originates from the maxillary bone, posterior-lateral to the inferior aspect of the posterior lacrimal crest.

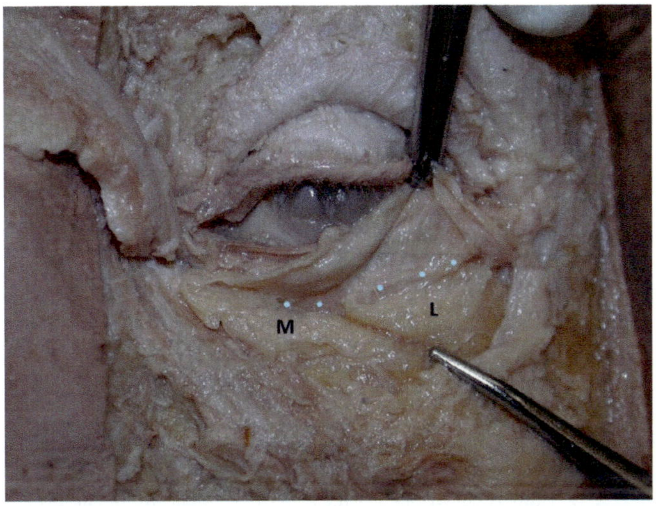

Fig. 3.15 The medial (M) and lateral (L) fat pads are divided by a fascial band (pointer) made of fibers from periorbita and orbital septum extending supramedially from the orbital rim to the capsulopalpebral fascia, often referred to as Lockwood's ligament (blue dots)

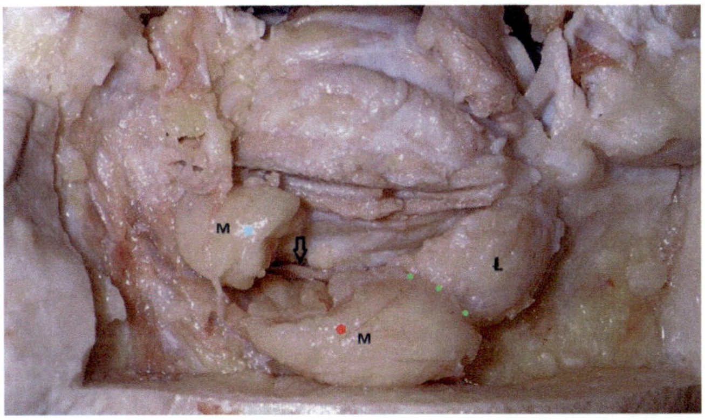

Fig. 3.16 Inferior oblique muscle (arrow) is dividing medial fat pad (M) into a nasal fat pad (blue dot) and central fat pad (red dot). Note the fascial band (green dots) separating the medial fat pad from the lateral fat pad (L)

Clinical correlation:

(a) Surgically, with this subdivision of the medial fat pad, the lower lid is considered to have three surgical fat pads: the nasal, central, and lateral fat pads.
(b) Care is taken during fat management to avoid injury to the inferior oblique muscle during lower lid blepharoplasty surgery.

Lower Lid Retractors

16. Together, the capsulopalpebral fascia and the inferior tarsal muscle are known as the lower lid retractors. Next, depress the orbital fat, and note lower lid retractors inserting on the inferior edge of the tarsus of the lower lid (Fig. 3.17).

The fibrous appearing band is that of the lower lid retractors, consisting of the fusion of the inferior tarsal muscle and the capsulpalpebral fascia (CPF). The CPF is an extension of the inferior rectus muscle after it wraps around the inferior obliquie muscle to extend toward the lower border of the tarsus of the lower lid.

Clinical correlation: Care is taken during central fat pad management to avoid injury to the inferior rectus muscle during lower lid blepharoplasty surgery.

The inner surface of the capsulopalpebral fascia is lined by smooth muscle known as the inferior tarsal muscle. It is difficult to identify in the cadaver.

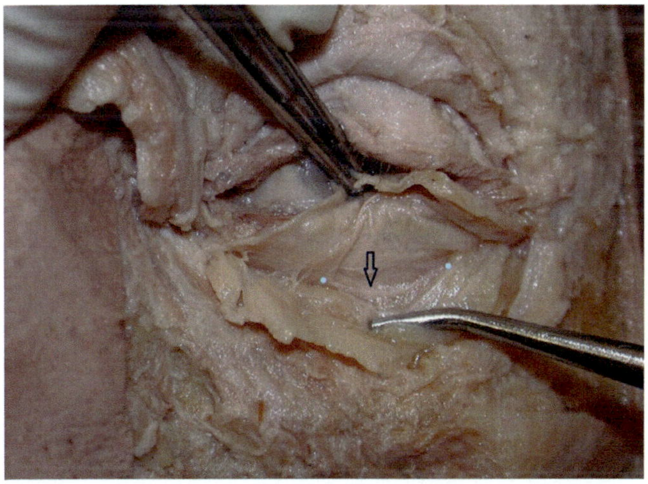

Fig. 3.17 The lower lid retractors (arrow) are seen as a white band. The septum of the lower lid is dissected from the arcus marginalis and reflected superiorly in the forceps but still attached to the lower lid retractors at the blue dots. The lower lid fat pads are reflected inferiorly by the pointer

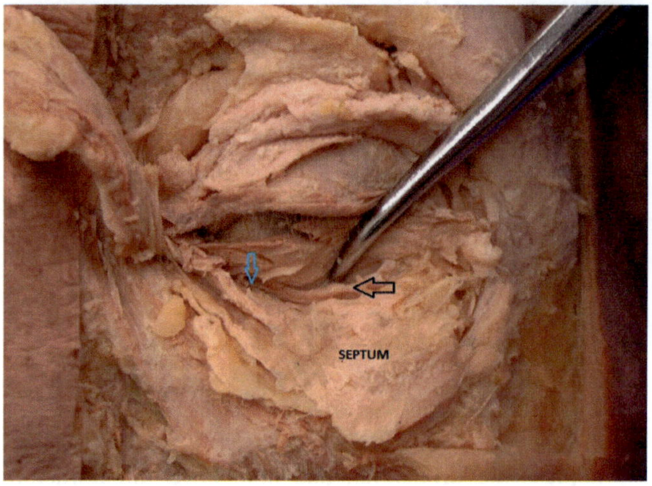

Fig. 3.18 The lower lid retractors are detached (black arrow) from the tarsus (pointer) going toward inferior oblique origin (blue arrow)

17. Incise and detach the retractors from the inferior edge of the lower tarsus (Fig. 3.18), leaving the inferior septum attached to the retractors.
18. Identify the inferior oblique muscle (*see* Fig. 3.16) and then dissect it to its origin.

    Note its relationship to the lower lid retractors. The inferior orbital fat may carefully be removed to enhance exposure.

    Lockwood's suspensory ligament is formed by conjoining of the:

- *Inferior oblique sheath.*
- *Inferior rectus sheath.*
- *Inferior portion of the interrectus muscle fascia.*
- *Lower lid retractors.*

Clinical correlation:

(a) Large inferior rectus muscle resections for strabismus surgery or inferior muscle entrapment in orbital floor fractures can result in lower lid retraction.

(b) Large recessions of the inferior rectus muscle for strabismus surgery or involutional disinsertions of the lower lid retractors can result in elevation of the lower lid margin.

(c) Disinsertion of the lower lid retractors is the anatomical factor in tarsal ectropion formation.

19. Perform a 360-degree conjunctival peritomy and identify the rectus muscle origins. Note their distance from the corneoscleral limbus.

Clinical correlation: The following measurements are helpful to the surgeon when performing strabismus surgery or enucleation surgery:

- Spiral of Tillaux:
- Medial rectus: 5.5 mm.
- Inferior rectus: 6.5 mm.
- Lateral rectus: 6.9 mm.
- Superior rectus: 7.7 mm.

Suggested Reading

Beard C, Quickert M. Anatomy of the Orbit. 2nd ed. Birmingham, AL: Aesculapius Publishing Company; 1977. p. 12–4.

Bedrossian EH Jr. Embryology and anatomy of the eyelid. In: Tasman W, Jaeger E, editors. Foundations of Clinical Ophthalmology, vol. 1. Philadelphia: Lippincott; 1998. p. 1–23.

Della Rocca RC, Bedrossian EH, Arthurs BP. Ophthalmic Plastic Surgery: Decision Making and Techniques. New York: McGraw Hill; 2002. p. 28–33.

Lemke B, Stasior O, Rosen P. The surgical relations of the levator palpebrae superioris muscle. Ophthal Plast Reconstr Surg. 1988;4:25–30.

Meyer D, Linberg J, Wobig J, McCormick S. Anatomy of the orbital septum and associated lid connective tissues: implication for ptosis surgery. Ophthal Plast Reconstr Surg. 1991;7:104–13.

4 Neuroanatomy: Cavernous Sinus

Edward H. Bedrossian, Jr

This chapter demonstrates removal of the orbital roof and exposure of the cavernous sinus, examining the structures within and providing clinical correlations.

The specimen has been cut horizontally above the brow (Fig. 4.1). A second cut is made at the base of the nose (Fig. 4.2), as per Chap. 1.

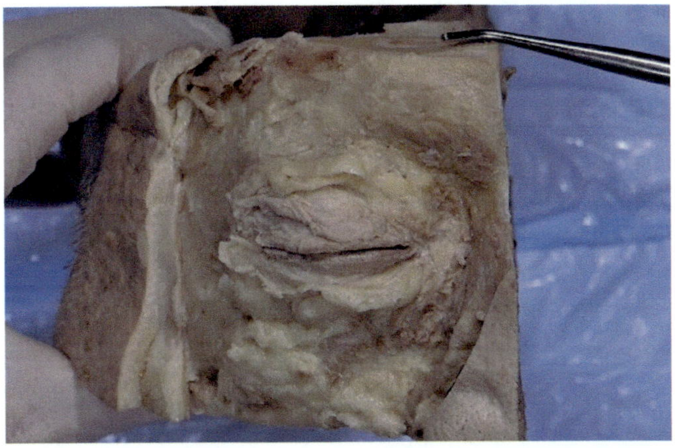

Fig. 4.1 The prepared specimen, indicating the location of the bone cut above the brow

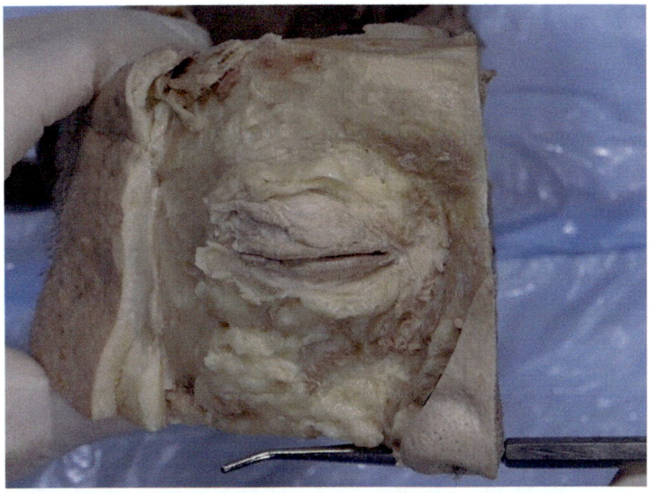

Fig. 4.2 The prepared specimen, indicating the location of the bone cut below the base of the nose

E. H. Bedrossian, Jr, MD, FACS (✉)
Wills Eye Hospital, Philadelphia, PA, USA

E. H. Bedrossian, Jr et al. (eds.), *Anatomy of the Eyelid, Orbit, and Lacrimal System*,
https://doi.org/10.1007/978-3-030-88265-5_4

Removal of the Orbital Roof

1. Carefully remove the frontal, temporal, and occipital lobes preventing damage to the brain stem (Figs. 4.3, 4.4, and 4.5). Note the frontal sinus (Fig. 4.6), roof of the orbit (Fig. 4.7), lateral wall of cavernous sinus within the middle cranial fossa (Fig. 4.8), olfactory bulb (Fig. 4.9), and intracanalicular optic nerve (Fig. 4.10).

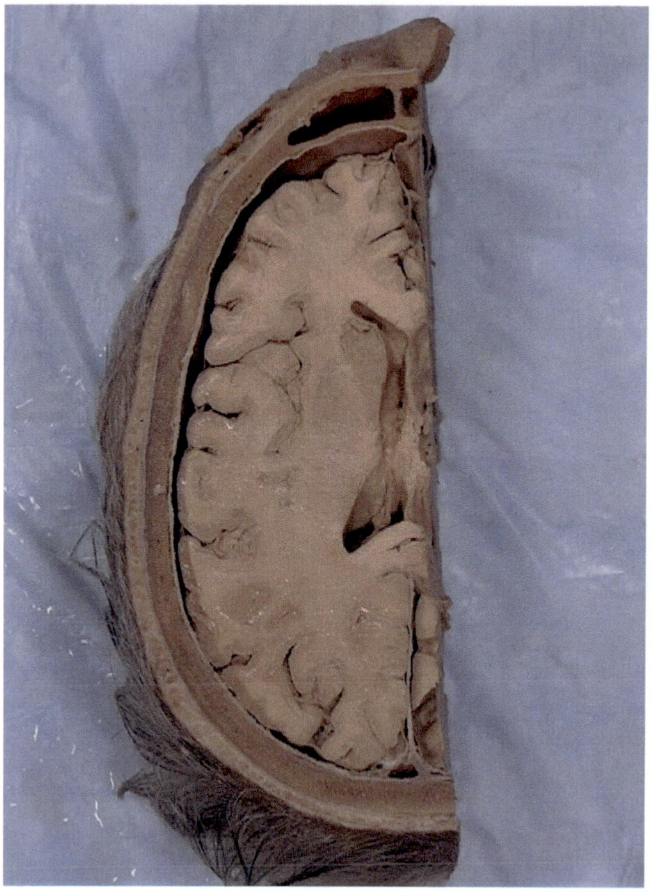

Fig. 4.3 View of specimen from above

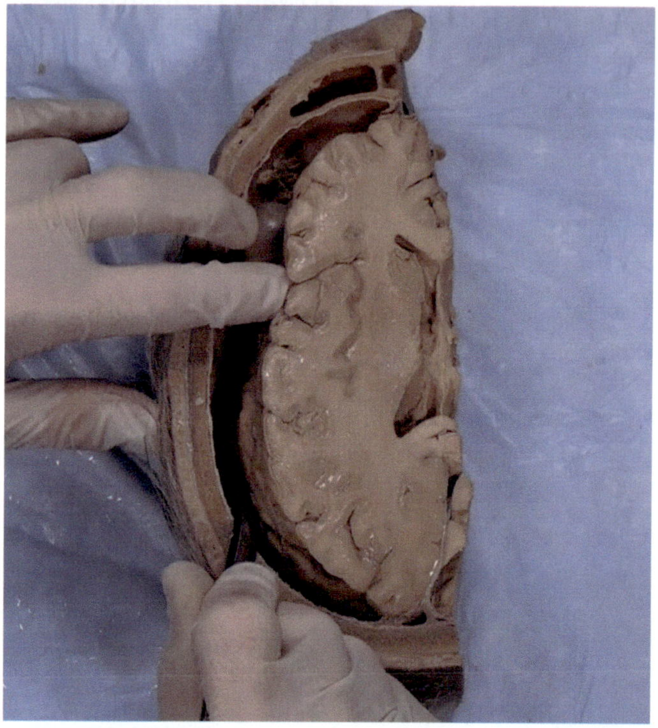

Fig. 4.4 Elevation of the frontal, temporal, and occipital lobes from the skull base

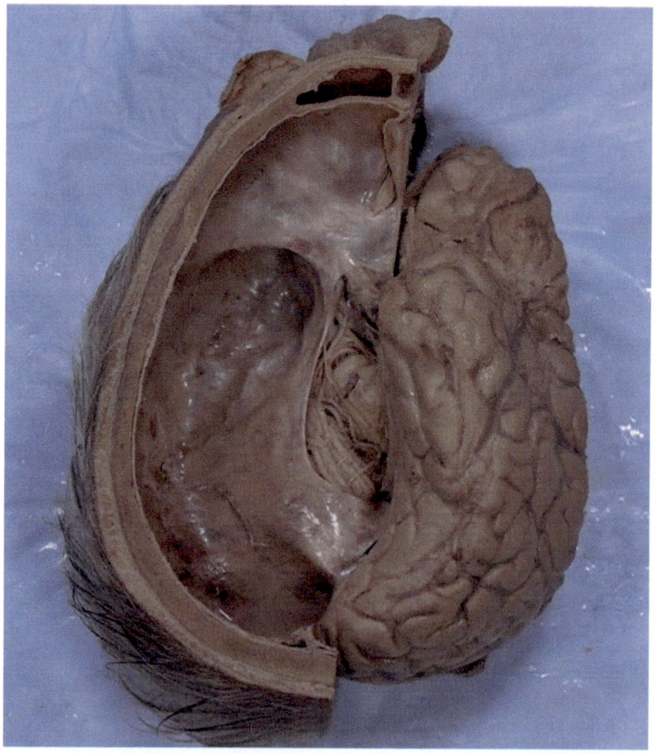

Fig. 4.5 Medially reflected brain, exposing the anterior, middle, and posterior cranial fossae

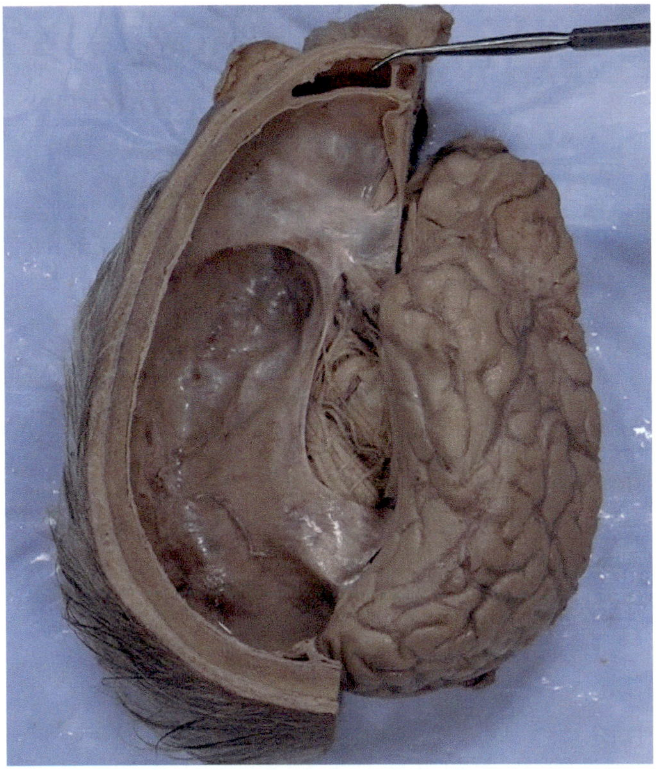

Fig. 4.6 The frontal sinus (pointer)

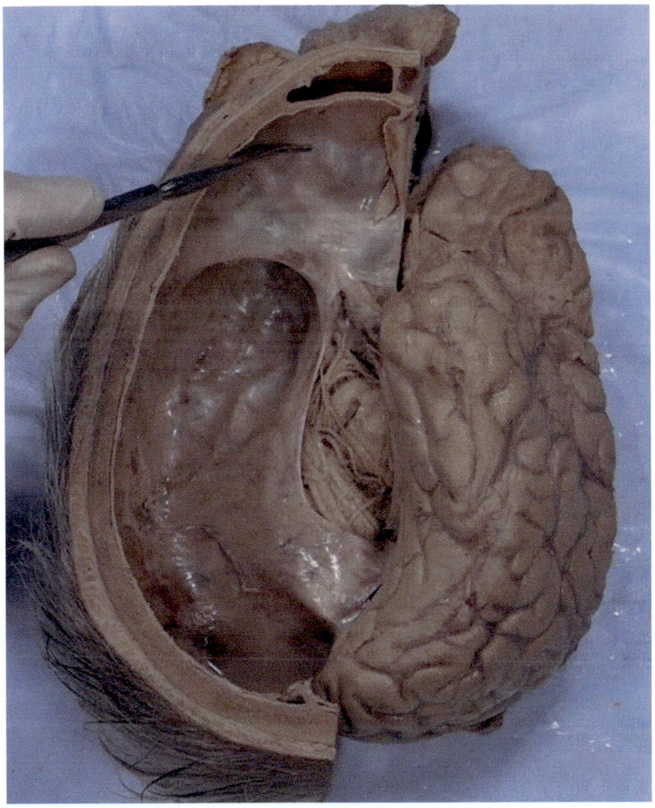

Fig. 4.7 The roof of the orbit (orbital plate of the frontal bone)

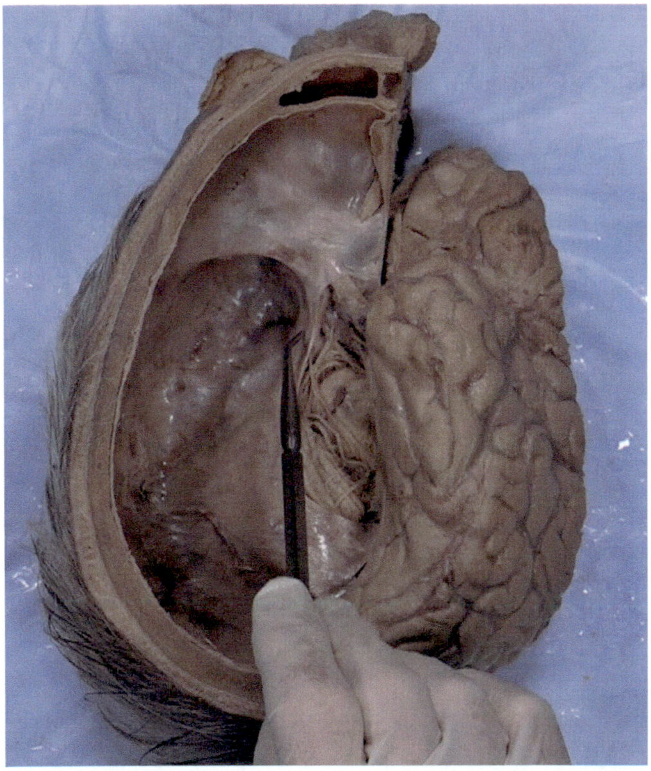

Fig. 4.8 Lateral wall of cavernous sinus (dura of middle cranial fossa)

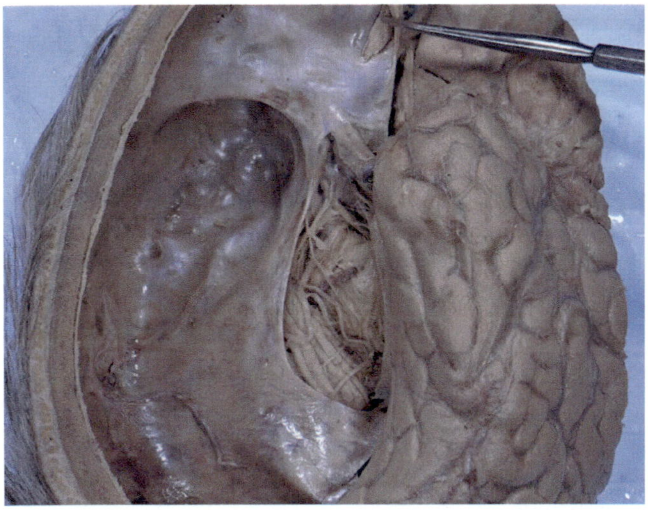

Fig. 4.9 Olfactory bulb

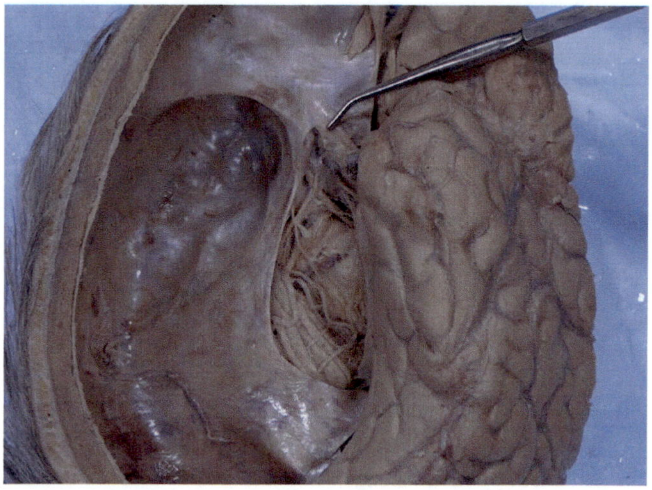

Fig. 4.10 Intracanalicular optic nerve

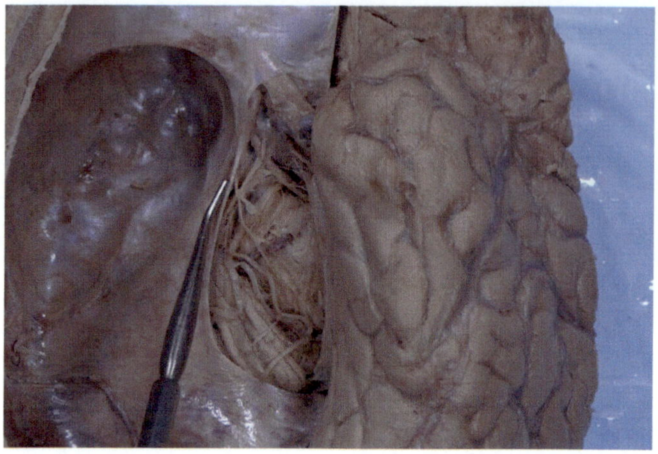

Fig. 4.12 The very delicate cranial nerve IV, trochlear nerve, entering the dura to assume the lateral-most position in the cavernous sinus

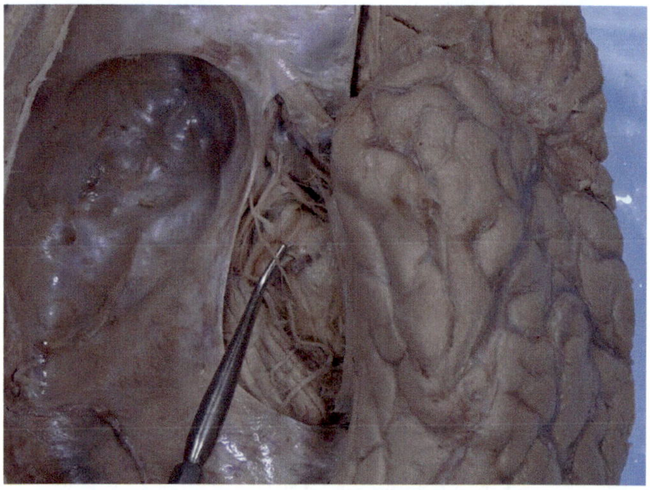

Fig. 4.11 The very delicate cranial nerve IV (trochlear nerve), arising dorsally from the midbrain

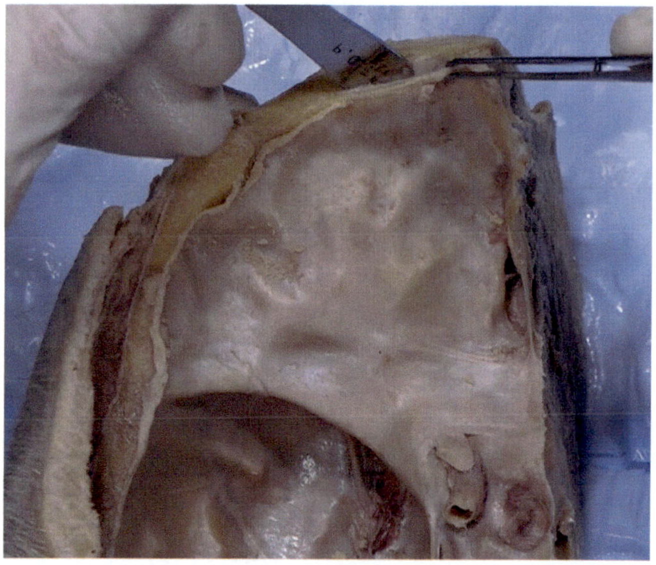

Fig. 4.13 Initial reflection of the dura from the frontal bone anteriorly

2. Identify the very delicate cranial nerve IV, trochlear nerve (Fig. 4.11), arising dorsally from the midbrain and entering the dura to assume the lateral-most position in the cavernous sinus (Fig. 4.12).

Clinical correlation: The trochlear nerve is unique among the cranial nerves because it is the only completely crossed cranial nerve and it is the only cranial nerve that exits the brain stem dorsally. The long and curved course of the trochlear nerve makes it prone to mechanical injury. Trochlear nerve palsy is sometimes seen in victims of traumatic head injury, causing superior oblique palsy. Lesion of the trochlear nerve leads to ocular skew deviation and diplopia. The brain compensates for the skew deviation by contralateral head tilt, called the Bielschowsky sign.

3. Clean the dura from the orbital roof (Figs. 4.13 and 4.14) to the optic canal.
4. Crack the orbital roof with an osteotome and mallet (Fig. 4.15). Then remove the bone piecemeal (Fig. 4.16).
5. Depress and separate the periorbita from the bone, anteriorly toward the orbital rim (Fig. 4.17).

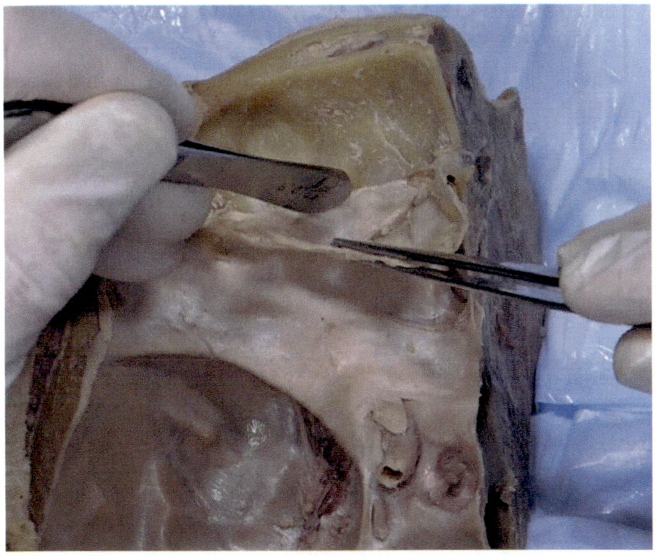

Fig. 4.14 Continued reflection of dura from the orbital roof

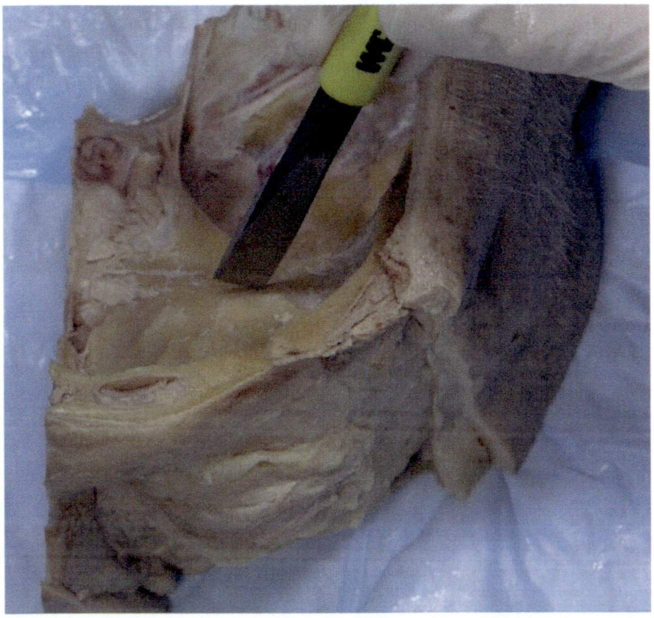

Fig. 4.15 Cracking of the orbital roof. This is facilitated by using the corner of the osteotome. The specimen is rotated 180 degrees

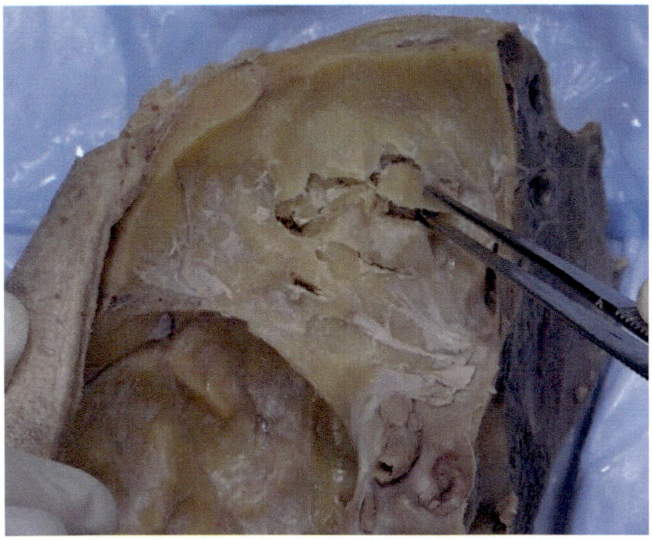

Fig. 4.16 Piecemeal removal of the orbital plate of the frontal bone exposing the periorbita

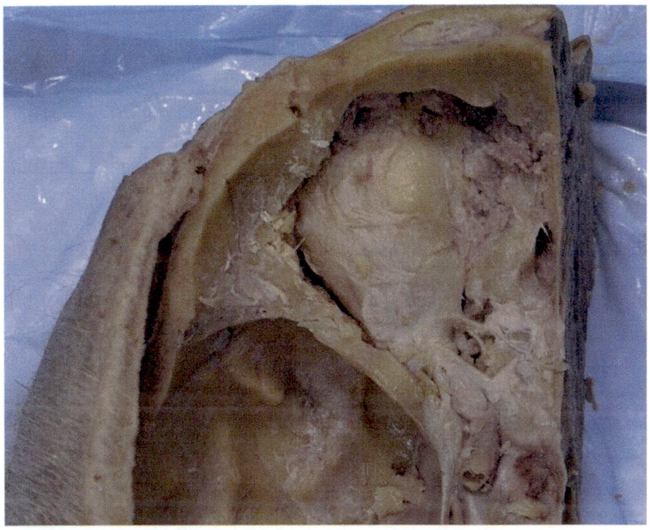

Fig. 4.17 The roof of the orbit removed, exposing the periorbital and orbital contents

6. Make two vertical cuts (Fig. 4.18), one through the frontal bone at the medial orbital border (Fig. 4.19) and a second at the lateral orbital border (Fig. 4.20). An osteotome and mallet can be used if a saw is unavailable. Care is taken not to cut too deeply as to disturb the soft tissue below.
7. Crack and anteriorly displace the isolated frontal bone fragment (Fig. 4.21).

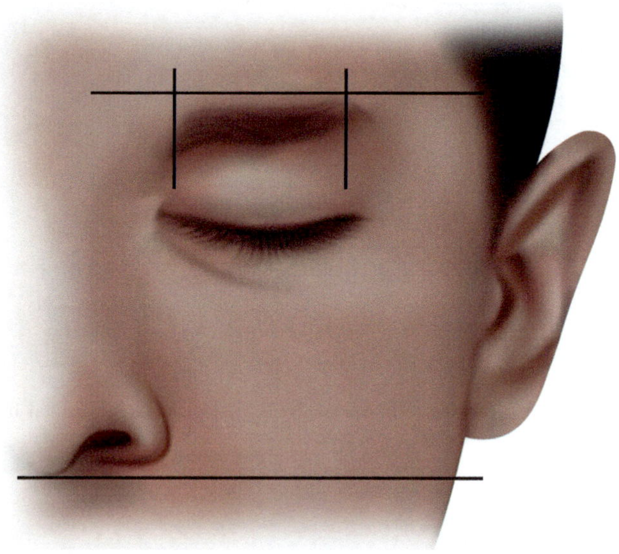

Fig. 4.18 Drawing showing location for medial and lateral vertical frontal bone cuts

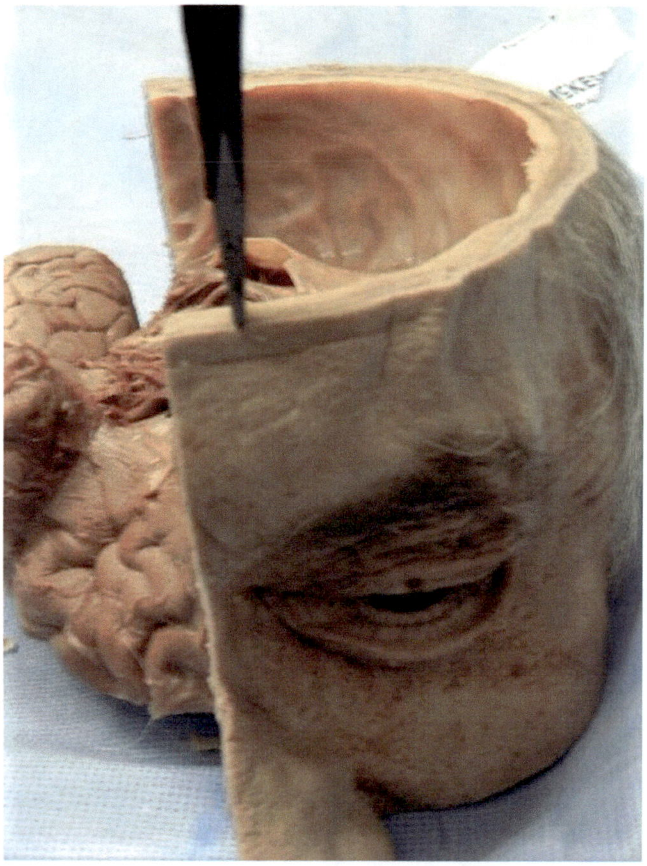

Fig. 4.19 Location of medial vertical frontal bone cut

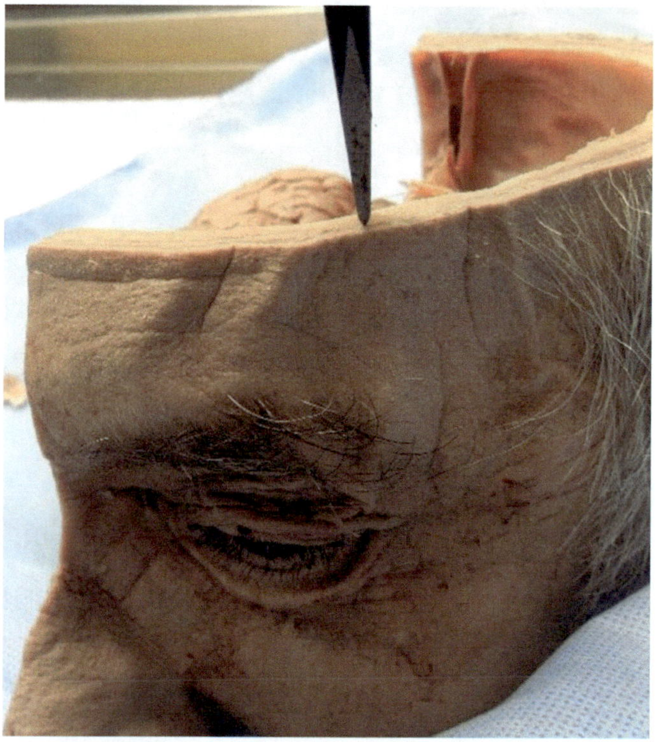

Fig. 4.20 Location of lateral vertical frontal bone cuts

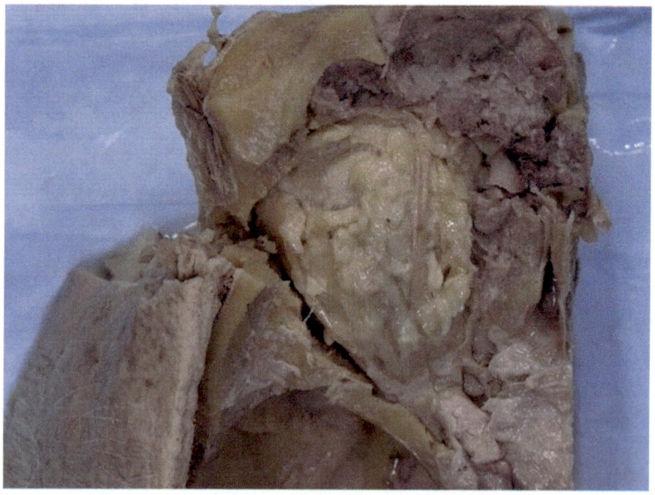

Fig. 4.21 Anteriorly displaced isolated frontal bone fragment

8. Note the supratrochlear nerve (Fig. 4.22) and, next to it, the supraorbital nerve (Fig. 4.23). If not seen deep to the periorbita, these two nerves will be further dissected in Chap. 5.

Clinical correlation: It is clear why supratrochlear and supraorbital nerve blocks for regional anesthesia of the medial and central portions of the upper eyelid are placed just inferior to the superior orbital rim.

9. Remove the isolated frontal bone fragment. You may need to cut the supratrochlear and supraorbital nerves.
10. Note the thin medial wall of the orbit and the ethmoid sinuses (Fig. 4.24).

Clinical correlations:

(a) The lamina papyracea is the thinnest of the orbital bones and is prone to fracture.
(b) Care must be taken during endoscopic medial wall decompression to avoid injury to the medial rectus muscle and other orbital structures.

11. Note the lateral wall of the orbit and its relationship to the middle cranial fossa (Fig. 4.25).

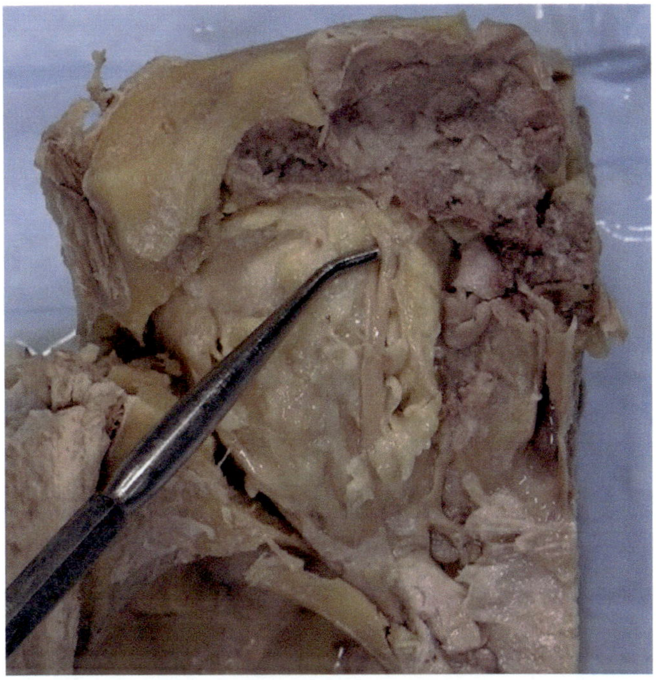

Fig. 4.22 The supratrochlear nerve

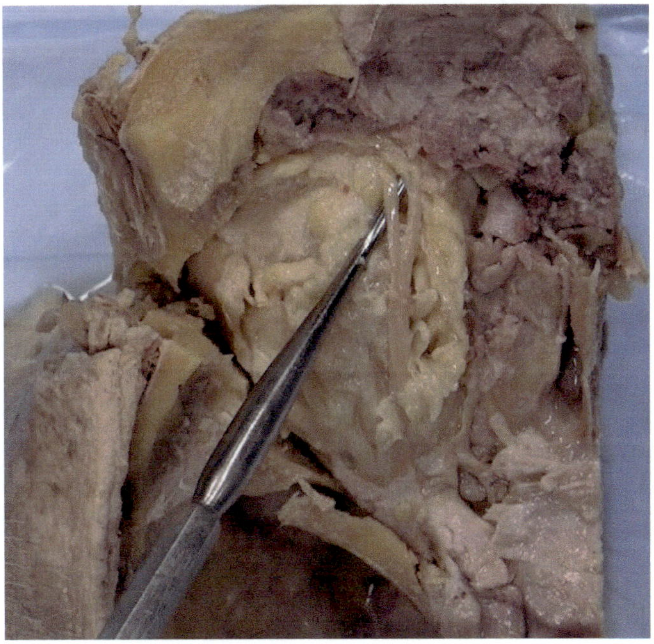

Fig. 4.23 The supraorbital nerve

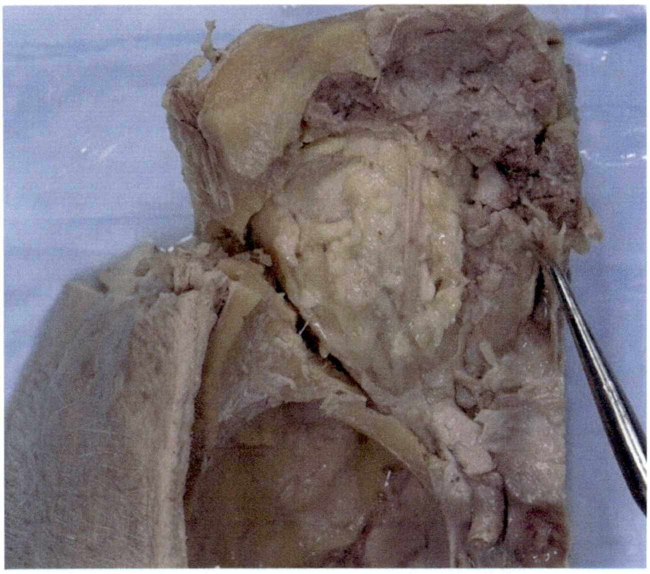

Fig. 4.24 The ethmoid sinuses medial to the medial wall of the orbit

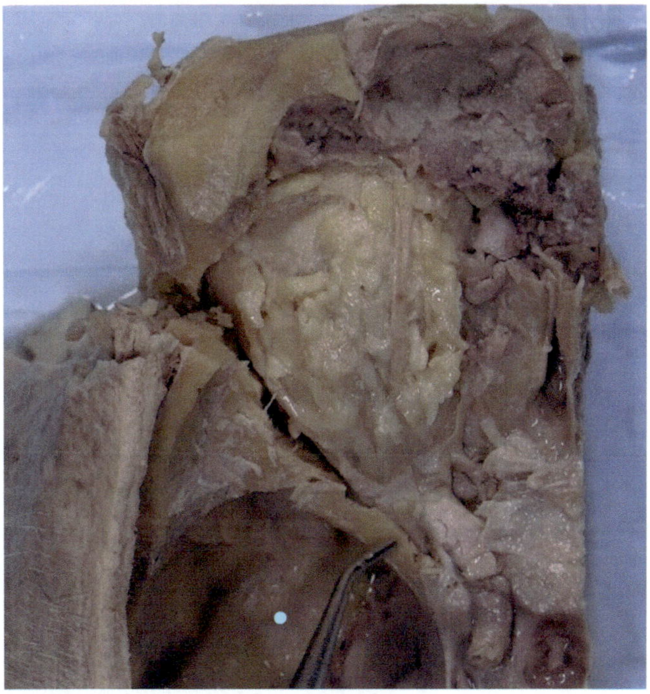

Fig. 4.25 The lateral wall of the orbit (pointer) and middle cranial fossa (blue dot)

Clinical correlation: These anatomic relationships are important when removing the bone during lateral wall decompressions.

Cavernous Sinus

12. Note the intracanalicular portion of the optic nerve (Fig. 4.26) and how the dura of the optic nerve is continuous with the periosteum.

Clinical correlation:

(a) Indirect traumatic optic neuropathy (TON) has been hypothesized to result from shearing injury to the intracanalicular portion of optic nerve, which can cause axonal injury or disturb the blood supply of the optic nerve. It has also been suggested that the optic nerve edema in the optic canal after trauma results in increased luminal pressure and secondary ischemic injury.

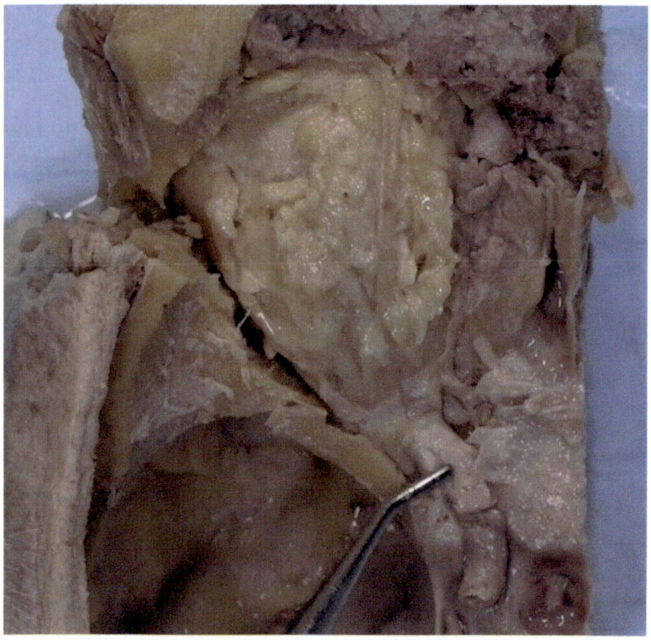

Fig. 4.26 The intracanalicular portion of the optic nerve

(b) Direct TON is presumed to be the result of tissue disruption secondary to foreign body or bony fragments impacting on the optic nerve.

13. Note the sagittal relationship of the optic chiasm (Fig. 4.27) to the sphenoid bone and sphenoid sinus (Fig. 4.28), carotid artery (Figs. 4.29 and 4.30), and pituitary gland and fossa (Fig. 4.31).

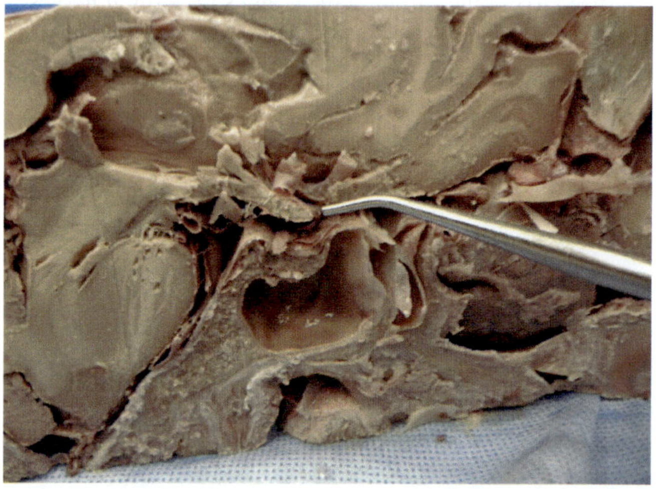

Fig. 4.27 The optic chiasm, sagittal view

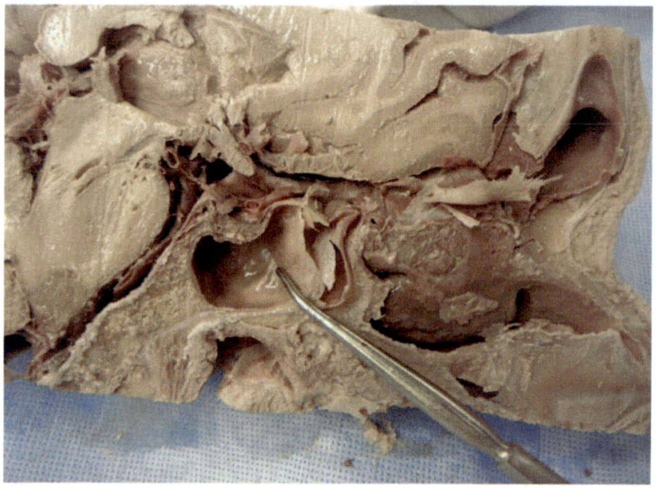

Fig. 4.28 The sphenoid sinus, sagittal view

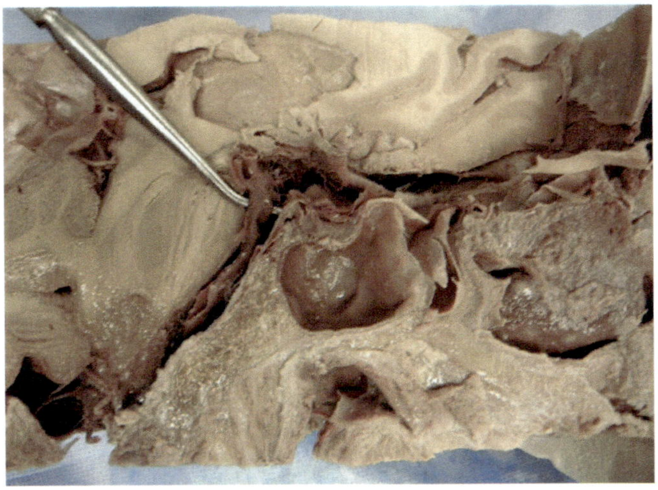

Fig. 4.29 The internal carotid artery

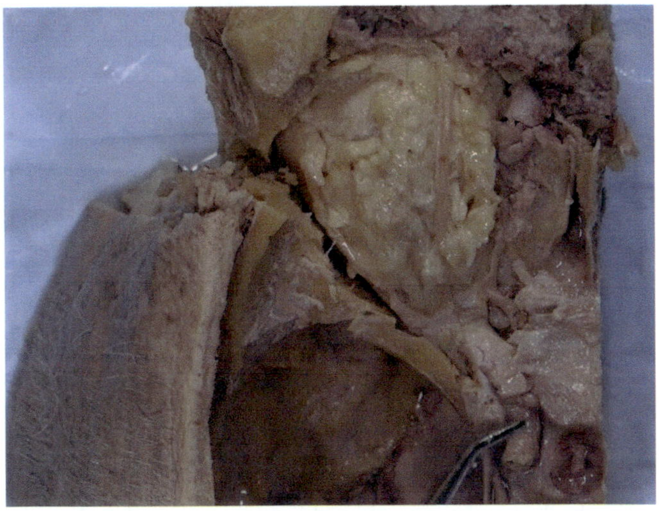

Fig. 4.30 The internal carotid artery in the unroofed cavernous sinus at orbital apex

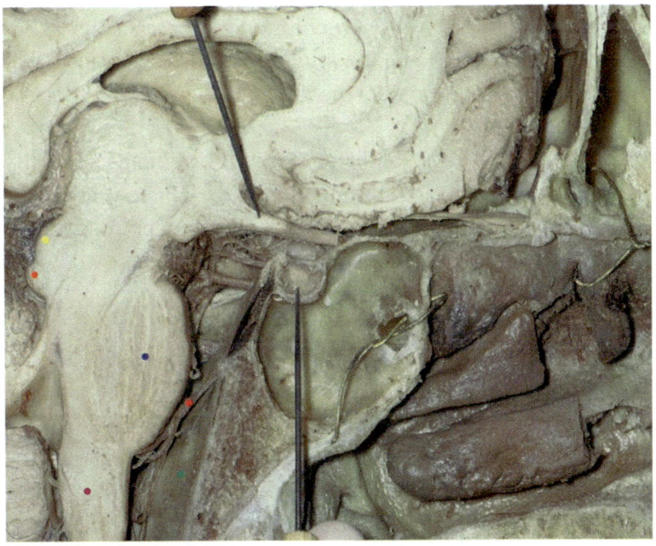

Fig. 4.31 Sagittal view of pituitary gland (lower pointer) within the pituitary fossa. Note the optic chiasm (superior pointer), superior colliculus (yellow dot), inferior colliculus (orange dot), pons (purple dot), medulla (magenta dot), clivus (green dot), and sixth nerve (red dot)

Clinical correlation:

(a) Large pituitary tumors compress the optic chiasm.
(b) Pituitary apoplexy with sudden bleeding into the tumor, severe headache, and visual disturbances is a medical emergency.

14. The cavernous sinus (Fig. 4.32) is a venous-filled space located on the lateral side of the body of the sphenoid bone. Its lateral wall is the dura of the middle cranial fossa (Fig. 4.33).
15. If not previously sacrificed when reflecting the brain stem, identify the very delicate cranial nerve IV, arising dorsally from the midbrain and entering the dura to assume the lateral-most position in the cavernous sinus (Figs. 4.11 and 4.12).

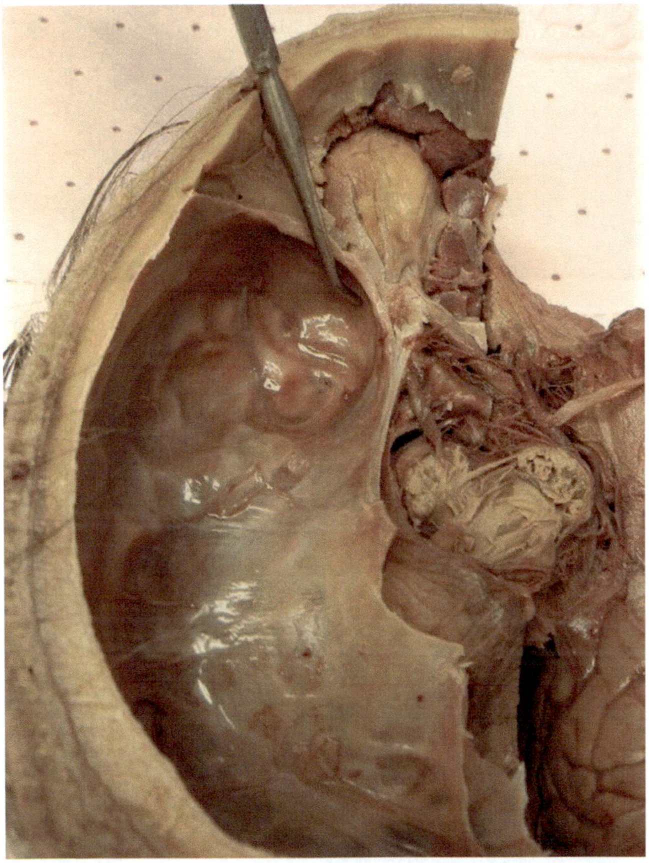

Fig. 4.32 The cavernous sinus (pointer) located on the lateral side of the body of the sphenoid bone

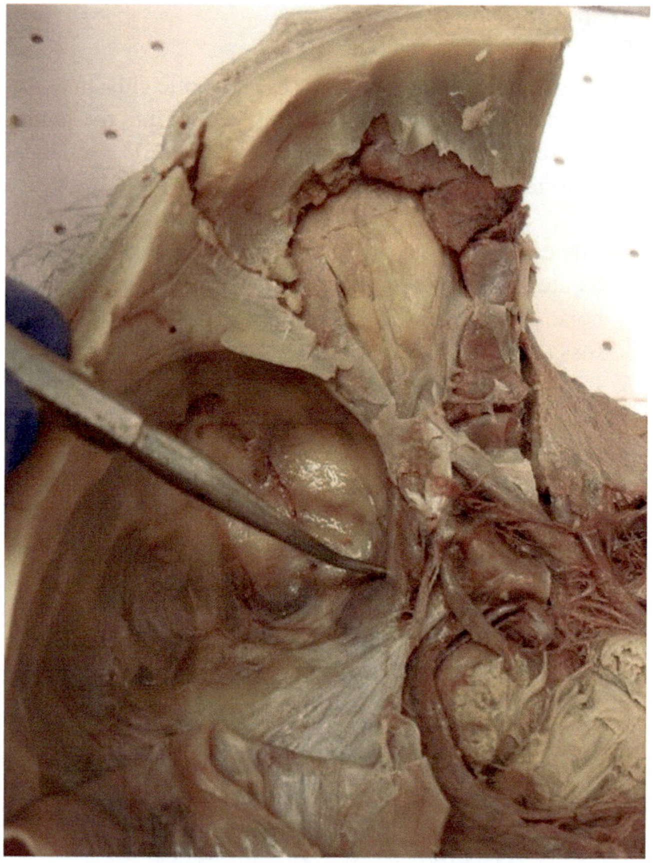

Fig. 4.33 The lateral wall of the cavernous sinus is the dura of the middle cranial fossa

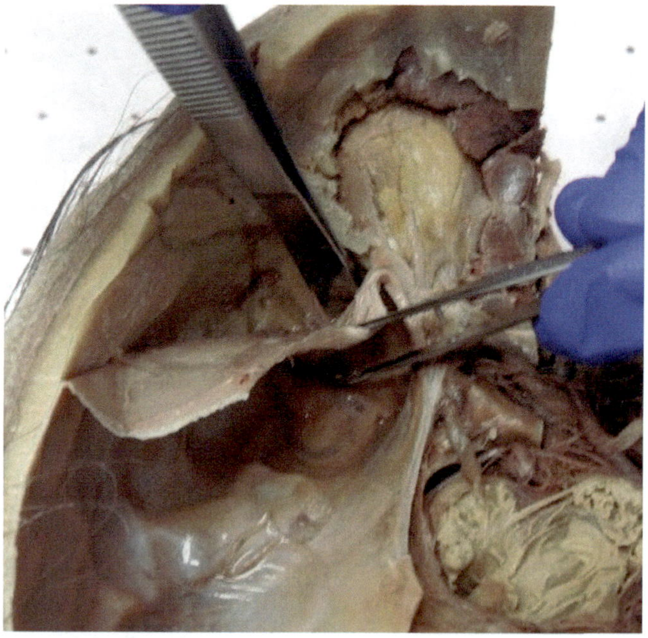

Fig. 4.34 Reflection of the dura of the middle cranial fossa, toward the cavernous sinus

16. Carefully elevate the dura of the middle cranial fossa and then the dura comprising the lateral wall of the cavernous sinus exposing the nerves and blood clot within the cavernous sinus (Fig. 4.34).

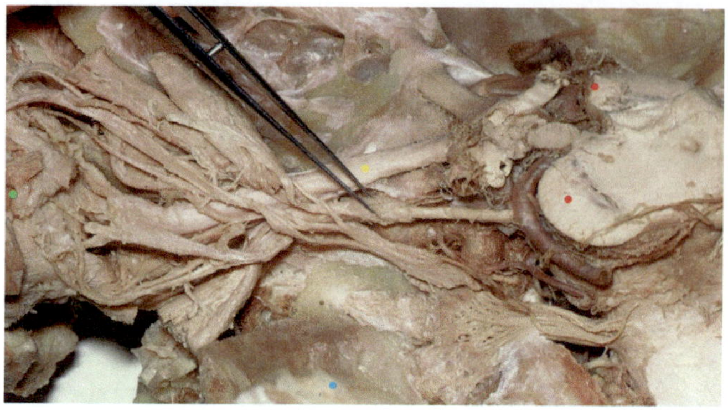

Fig. 4.35 Cranial nerve III (in forceps) in cavernous sinus. Note the superior colliculi (red dots) of the midbrain, orbit (green dot), middle cranial fossa (blue dot), and optic nerve (yellow dot)

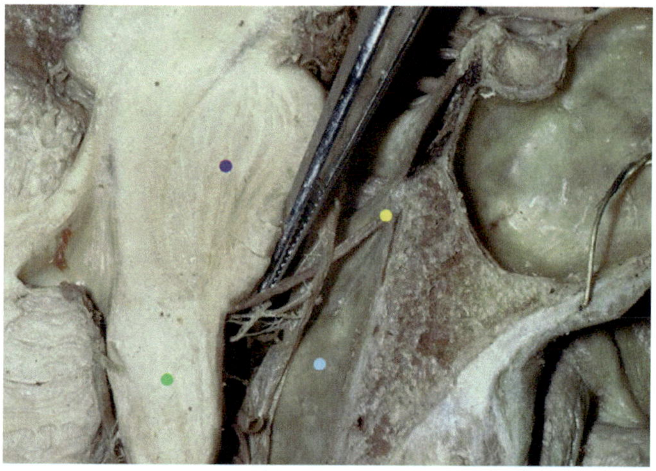

Fig. 4.36 Cranial nerve VI (abducens nerve) originates ventrally from the pons-medulla junction (pointer), ascends the clivus (blue dot), and enters the dura at the petrosphenoid ligament (yellow dot). Note the pons (purple dot) and the medulla (green dot)

17. The cranial nerve III (oculomotor nerve) (Fig. 4.35) arises ventrally from the midbrain at the oculomotor sulcus and likewise enters the dura before reaching the cavernous sinus.
18. Cranial nerve VI (abducens nerve) originates ventrally from the pons-medulla junction (Fig. 4.36), ascends the clivus, and enters the dura at the petrosphenoid ligament.

Clinical correlation: The sixth nerve with its long tight course against the clivus is prone to decompressive injury, skull base fractures, and small vessel disease.

19. The multiple roots of cranial nerve V condense at the Gasserian ganglion (Figs. 4.37 and 4.38) and then course anteriorly. The ophthalmic and maxillary divisions both pass through the cavernous sinus.

Clinical correlation: Patients may present with similar signs and symptoms consistent with the orbital apex syn-

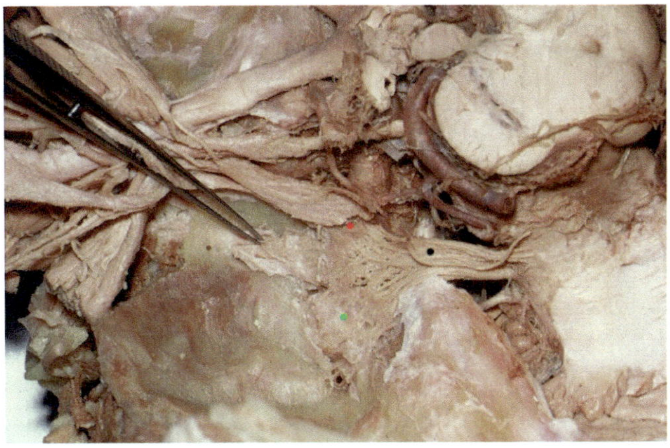

Fig. 4.37 The multiple roots of cranial nerve V condense at the Gasserian ganglion (black dot). The ophthalmic (red dot) and maxillary (pointer at foramen rotundum) divisions pass through the cavernous sinus. Note the mandibular division (green dot) passing through the foramen ovale and is outside the cavernous sinus

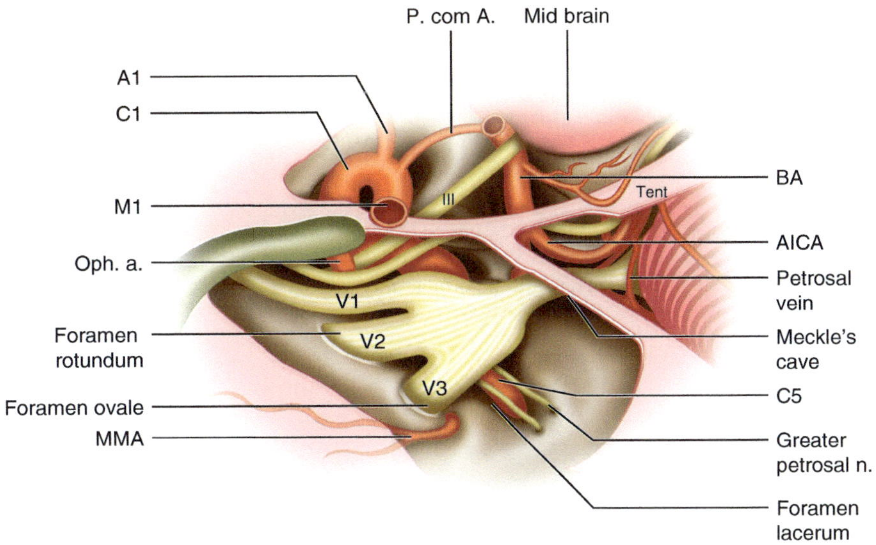

Fig. 4.38 Drawing of the cavernous sinus

drome, the superior orbital fissure, or the cavernous sinus syndrome. Clinical evaluation holds key to the differential diagnosis. Patients with cavernous sinus syndrome may note decreased sensation to the maxillary division of the trigeminal nerve. Those with orbital apex syndrome will have normal maxillary function.

20. Note that the medial wall of the cavernous sinus is the bone of the body of the sphenoid.

Suggested Reading

Beard C, Quickert M. Anatomy of the orbit. second ed. Birmingham, AL: Aesculapius Publishing Company; 1977. p. 23–6. 44, 56

Della Rocca RC, Bedrossian EH, Arthurs BP. Ophthalmic plastic surgery: decision making and techniques. New York: McGraw Hill; 2002. p. 212–8.

Korchi AM, Cuvinciuc V, Caetano J, Becker M, Lovblad KO, Vargas MI. Imaging of the cavernous sinus lesions. Diagn Interv Imaging. 2014;95(9):849–59.

Levin LA, Beck RW, Joseph MP, Seiff S, Kraker R. The treatment of traumatic optic neuropathy: the international optic nerve trauma study. Ophthalmol. 1999;106(7):1268–77.

Netter F. Atlas of human anatomy. sixth ed. Philadelphia: Saunders/Elsevier; 2014. p. 55, 73, 87, 104, 105, 149.

The Orbit: Superior Approach

5

Edward H. Bedrossian, Jr

In this chapter, dissection of the orbit will continue from a superior approach. First, the periorbita will be opened, and the structures above the muscle cone will be dissected. Then the levator and superior rectus muscles will be dissected, transected, and reflected, to enter the muscle cone. Next, structures within the muscle cone will be carefully dissected and identified. Clinical correlation will be provided.

Superior Orbit

1. Identify the periorbita by "tenting" it superiorly with forceps (Fig. 5.1). Longitudinally incise (Figs. 5.2 and 5.3), elevate (Figs. 5.4 and 5.5), and remove the *periorbita* (Fig. 5.6).

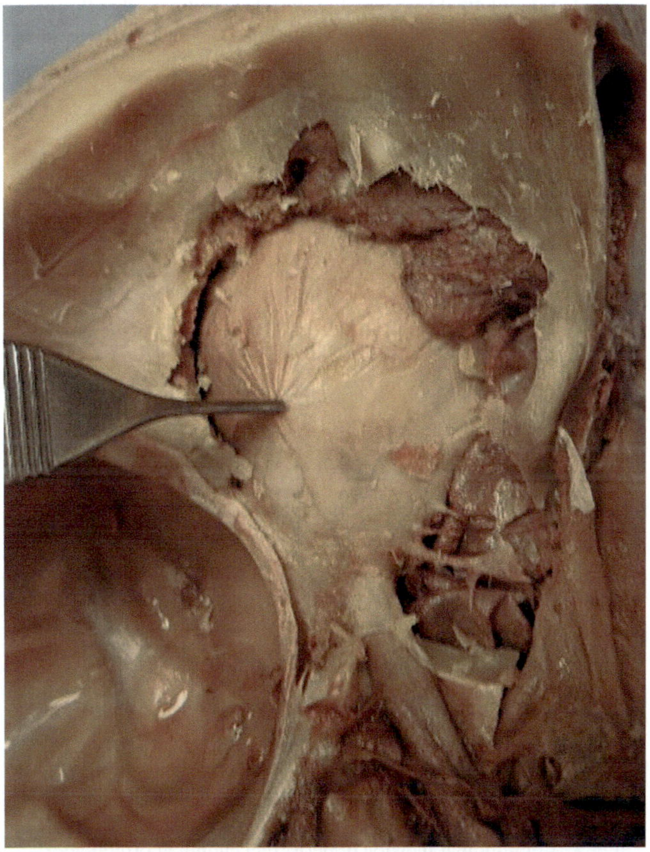

Fig. 5.1 The periorbita "tented" superiorly in forceps

E. H. Bedrossian, Jr, MD, FACS (✉)
Wills Eye Hospital, Philadelphia, PA, USA

E. H. Bedrossian, Jr et al. (eds.), *Anatomy of the Eyelid, Orbit, and Lacrimal System*,
https://doi.org/10.1007/978-3-030-88265-5_5

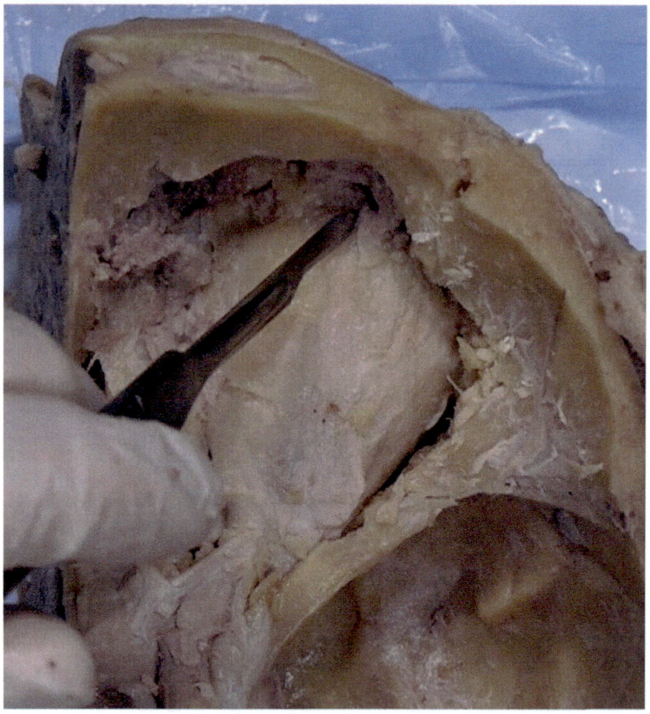

Fig. 5.2 Longitudinal incision of periorbita starting anteriorly

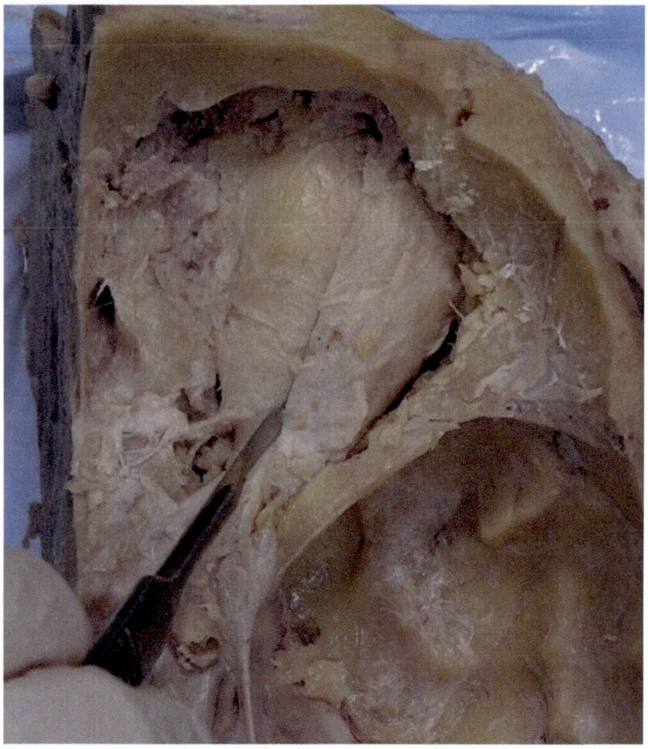

Fig. 5.3 Longitudinal incision of periorbita ending at orbital apex

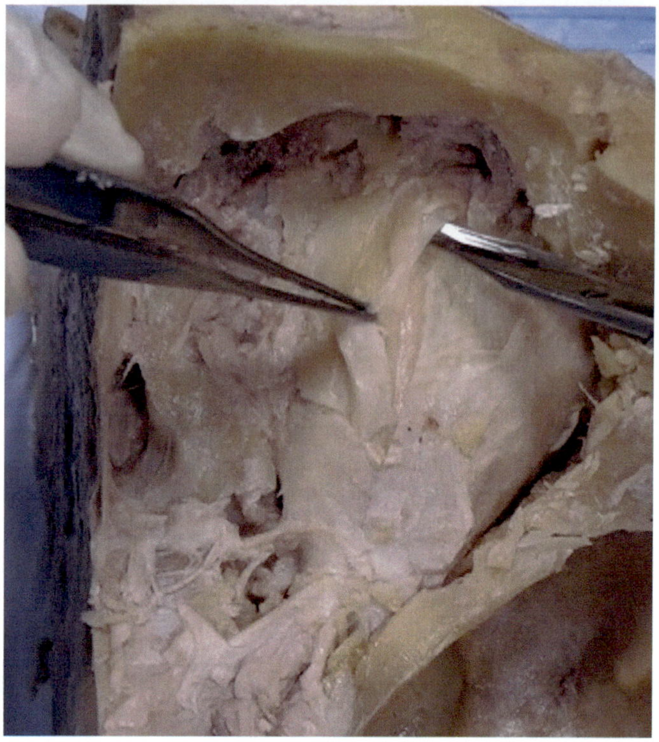

Fig. 5.4 Central and medial elevation of periorbita

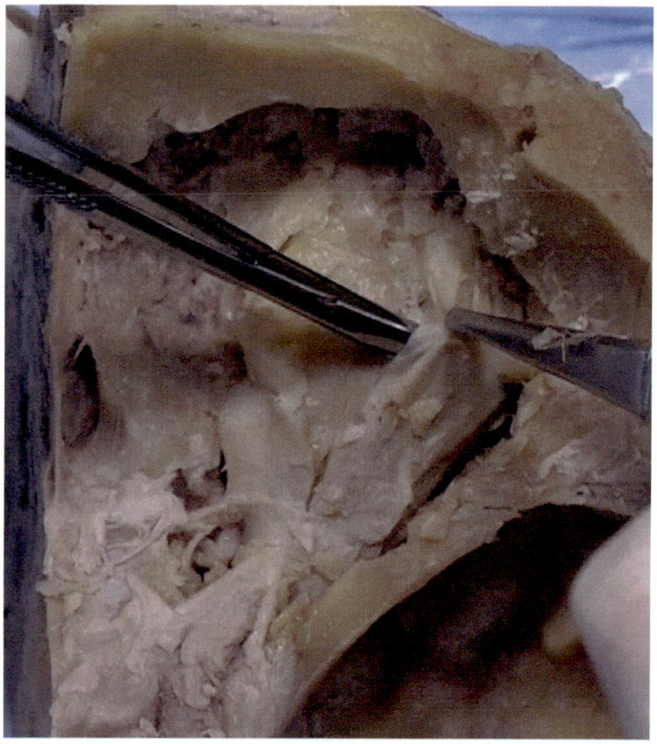

Fig. 5.5 Lateral elevation of periorbita

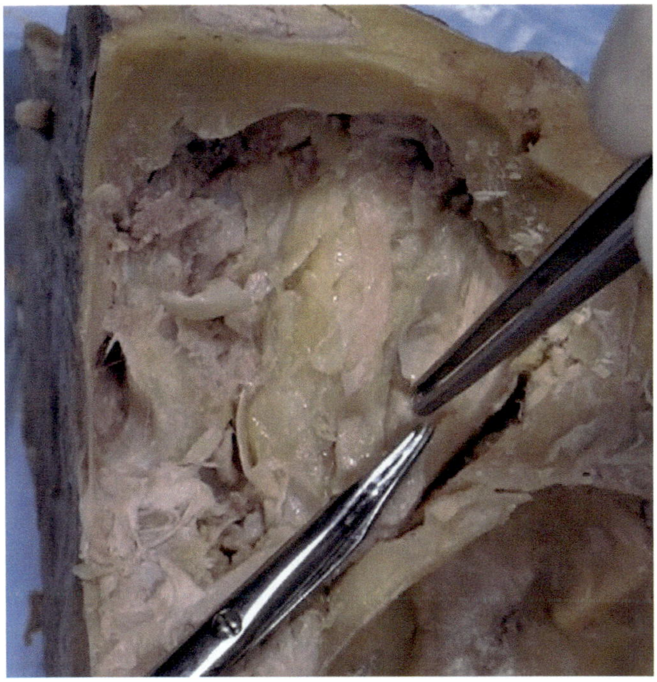

Fig. 5.6 Excision of periorbita along lateral orbital wall

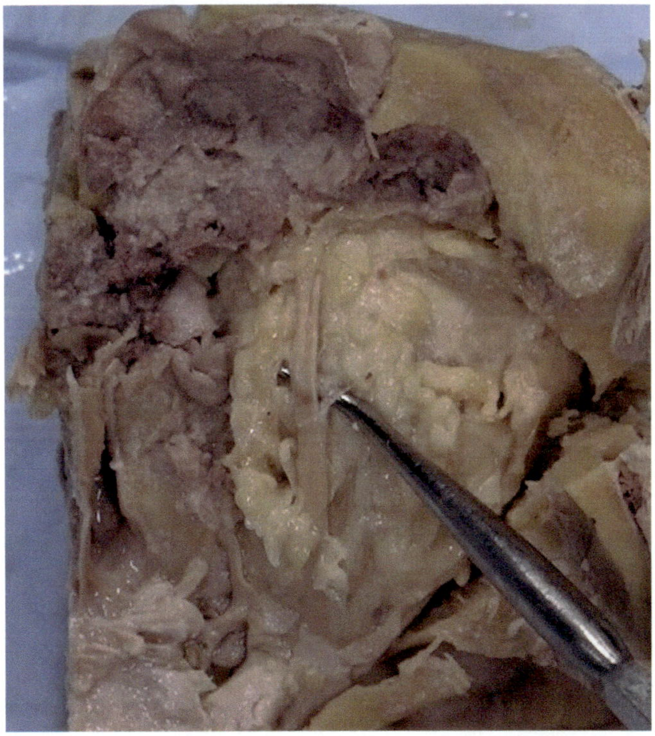

Fig. 5.7 The frontal nerve

2. Note the *frontal nerve* (Figs. 5.7 and 5.8) branching to form the *supraorbital* (Fig. 5.9) and *supratrochlear* (Fig. 5.10) *nerves*.

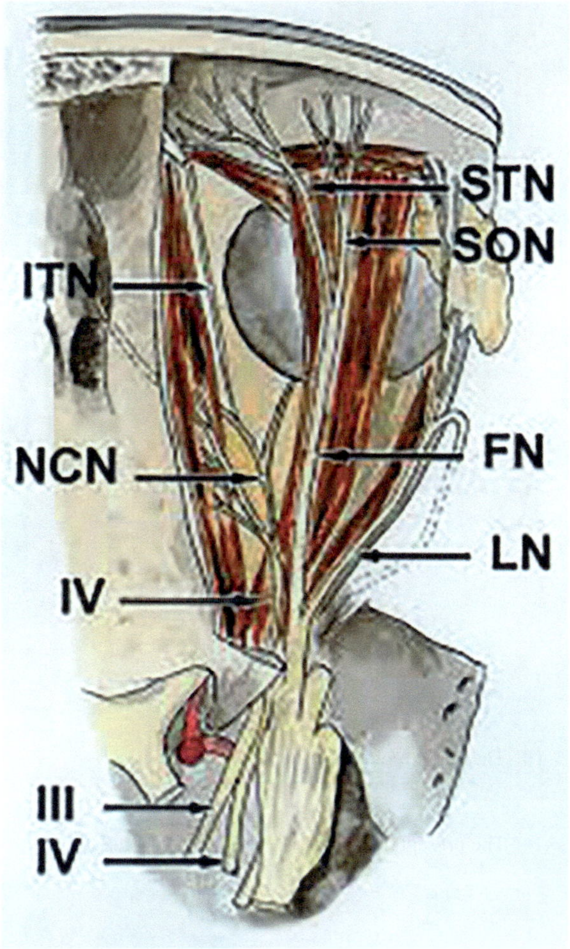

Fig. 5.8 Orbital nerves

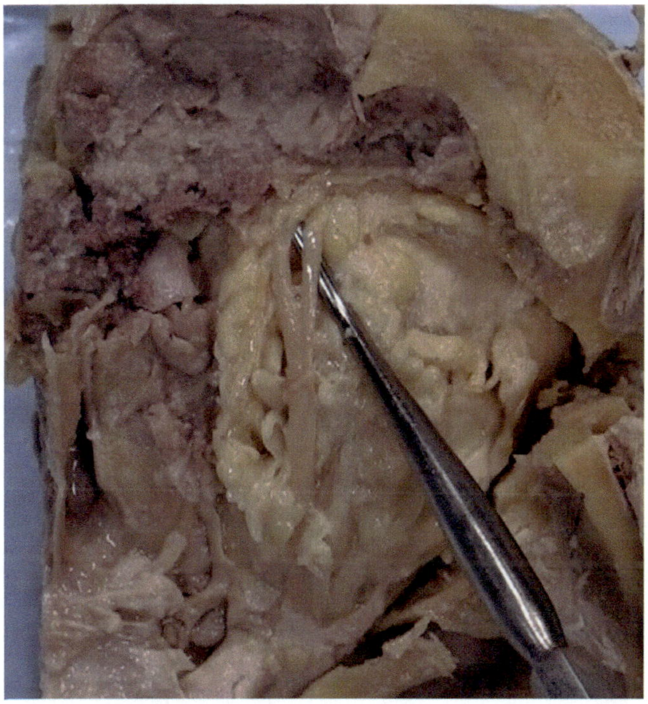

Fig. 5.9 The supraorbital nerve

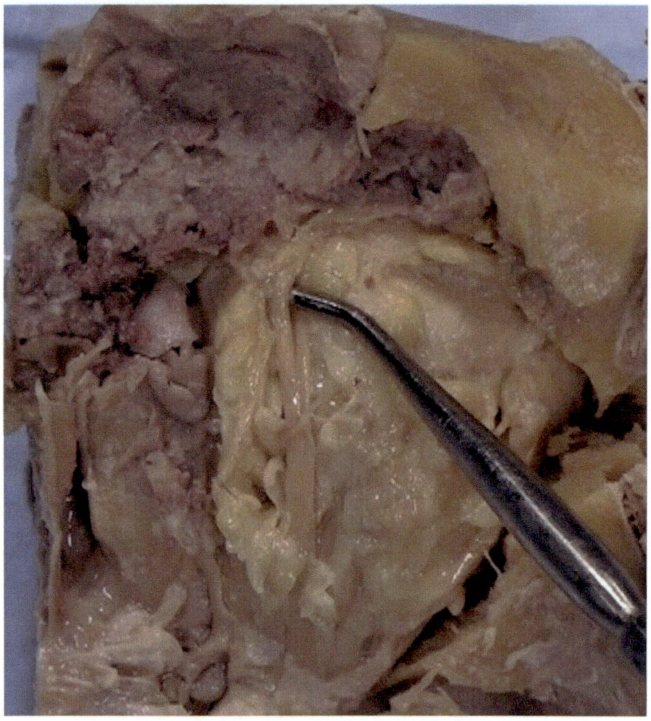

Fig. 5.10 The supratrochlear nerve

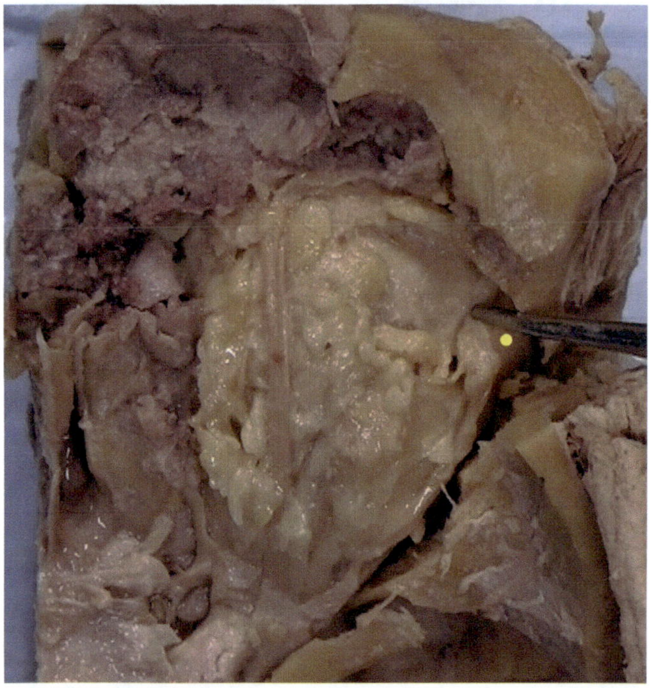

Fig. 5.11 The lacrimal gland below pointer (yellow dot)

3. Note the lacrimal gland (Fig. 5.11). The *lacrimal nerve* and *trochlear nerve* will be identified later.

Clinical correlation: From this viewpoint, it is clear why a frontal nerve block is made as superiorly in the orbit as possible.

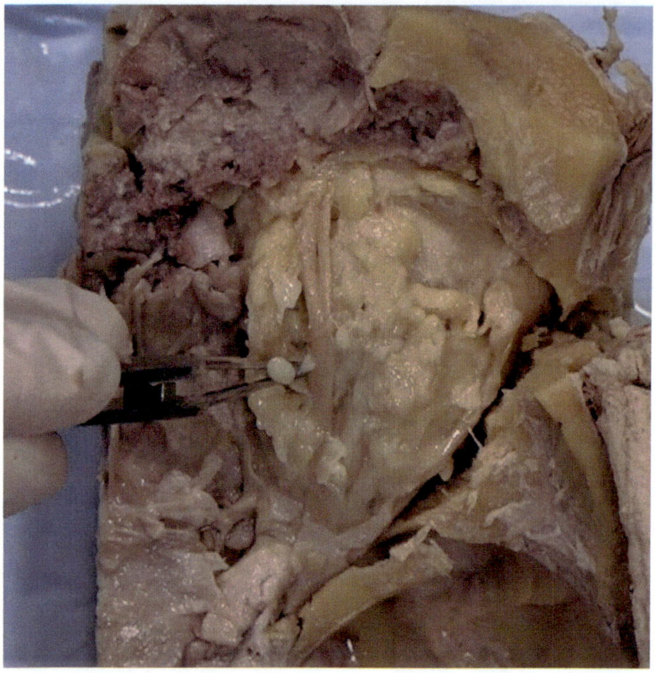

Fig. 5.12 Removal of superior orbital fat, in forceps

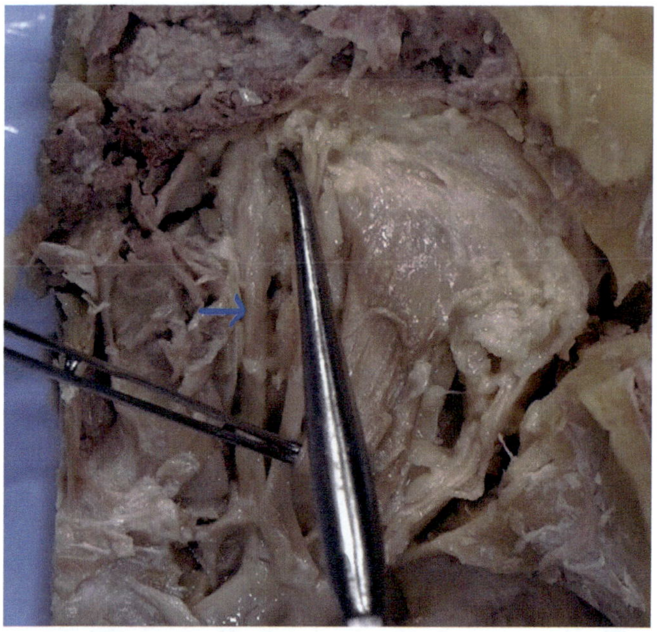

Fig. 5.13 The superior oblique muscle (arrow). Anteriorly, the pointer is on the trochlea

4. Carefully pick away the orbital fat (Fig. 5.12) to expose the *superior oblique muscle* (Fig. 5.13), tracing it only as far anteriorly as the trochlea.
5. Identify the supraorbital artery (Figs. 5.14, 5.15, and 5.16), supratrochlear artery (Figs. 5.14, 5.15, and 5.16), dorsal nasal artery (Fig. 5.17), and lacrimal artery (Fig. 5.16). They may be difficult to identify *without* dye injections.

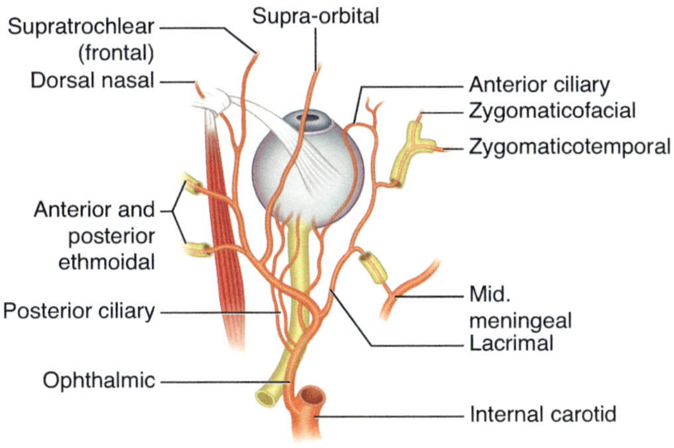

Fig. 5.14 Arterial supply to orbit

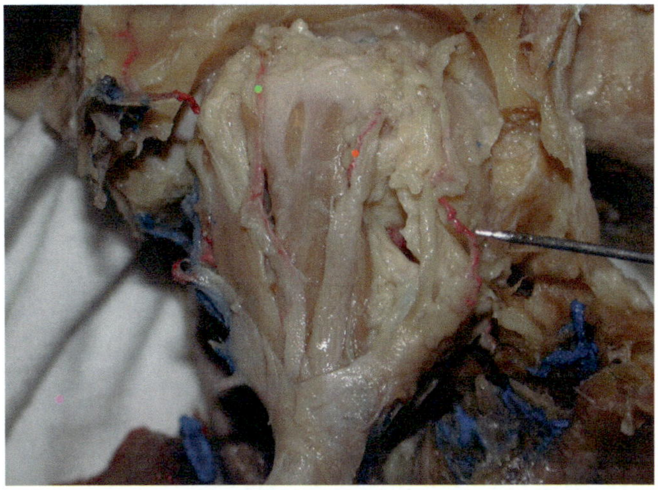

Fig. 5.15 The lacrimal artery (pointer). Note the supratrochlear artery (green dot) and the supraorbital artery (orange dot)

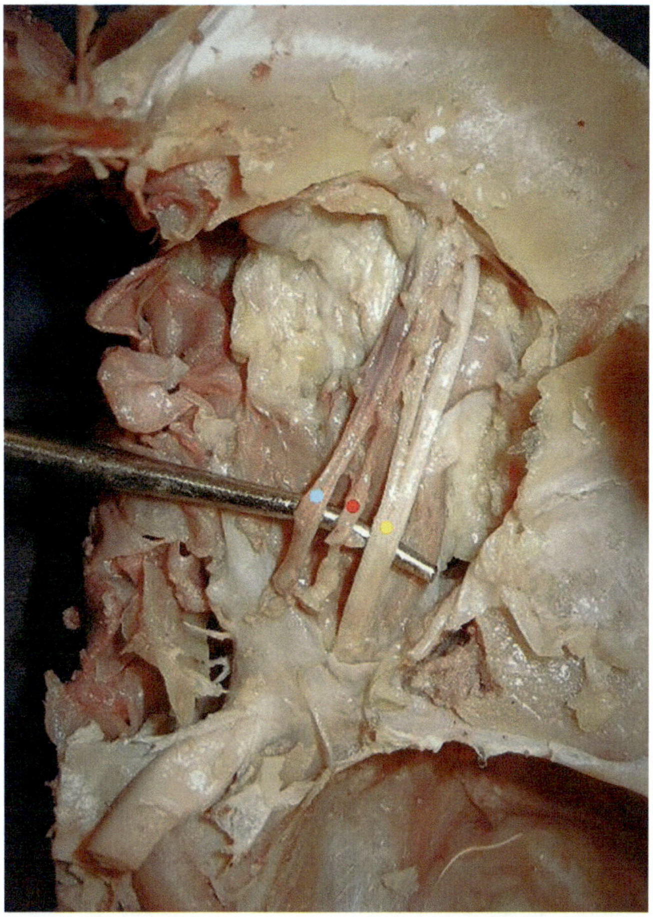

Fig. 5.16 The frontal nerve (yellow dot), supraorbital artery (red dot), and supraorbital vein (blue dot)

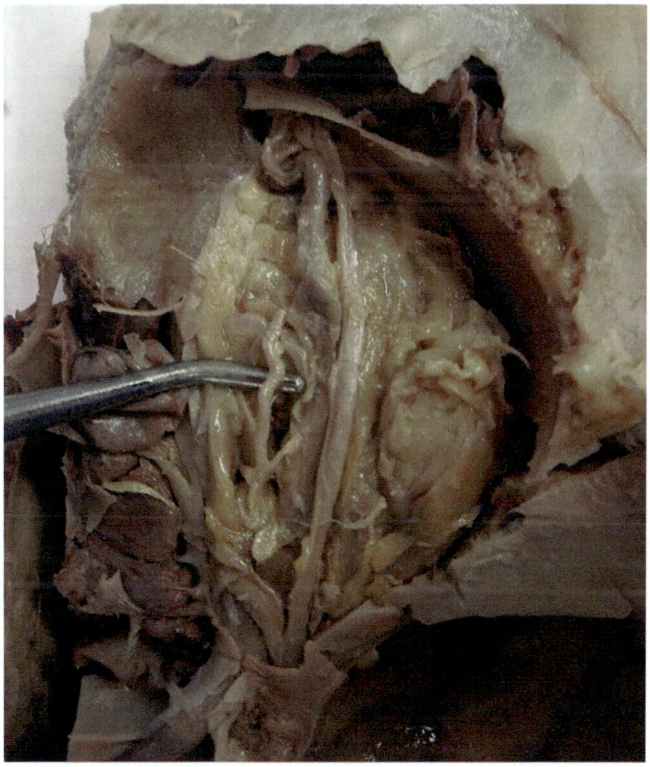

Fig. 5.17 Dorsal nasal artery

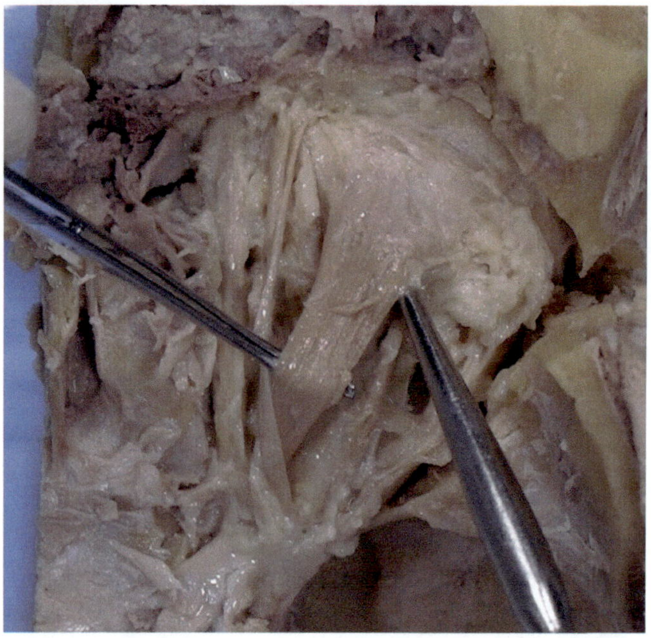

Fig. 5.18 The levator muscle

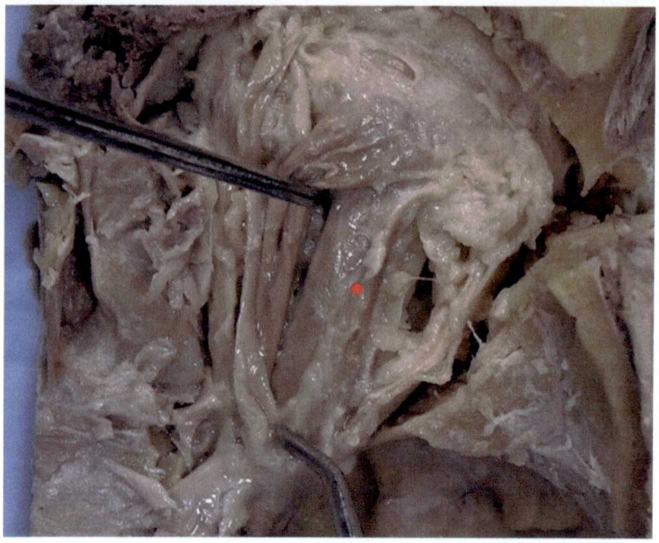

Fig. 5.20 The levator muscle is reflected in superior pointer, and the inferior pointer is at the annulus of Zinn, exposing the superior rectus muscle (red dot)

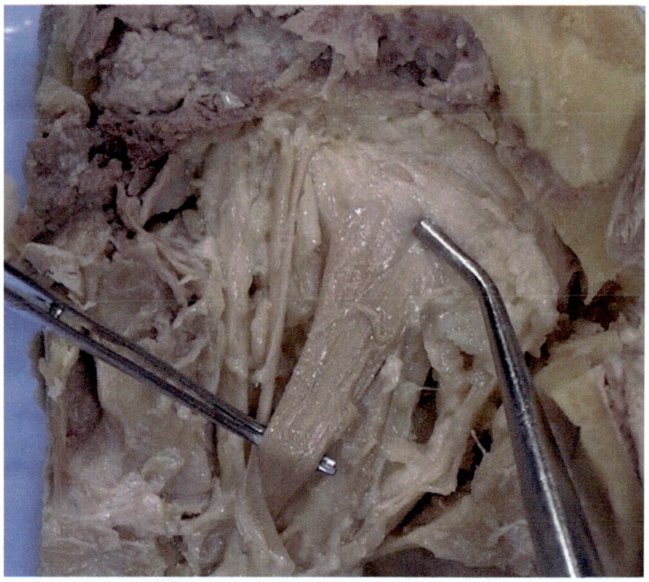

Fig. 5.19 Whitnall's ligament (pointer)

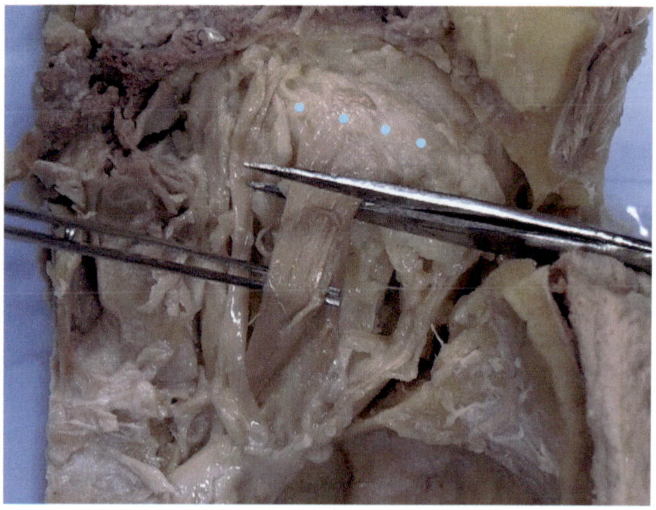

Fig. 5.21 The levator muscle within the scissors, posterior to Whitnall's ligament (blue dots)

6. Identify the *levator muscle* (Fig. 5.18). Note the anterior expansion of the levator muscle as it fans out into the fibrous aponeurosis. At this point, *Whitnall's ligament* traverses the muscle as a white-gray band (Fig. 5.19).
7. Reflect the levator muscle to expose the underlying *superior rectus muscle* (Fig. 5.20).
8. Cut the levator muscle 5 mm posterior to Whitnall's ligament (Figs. 5.21 and 5.22), and reflect it (Fig. 5.23), noting the insertion of the nerve to the levator muscle (third

nerve). Does the superior ramus of the oculomotor nerve (serving both the superior rectus muscle and the levator) pass around the superior rectus or through it?

9. Anteriorly, separate the fibrous attachments of superior rectus muscle from the undersurface of the levator muscle (Fig. 5.24).

Clinical correlation: Lysis of these fibrous attachments between the levator muscle and superior rectus muscle at the time of superior rectus bridle suture placement for anterior segment surgery may be a source of new onset post-op ptosis.

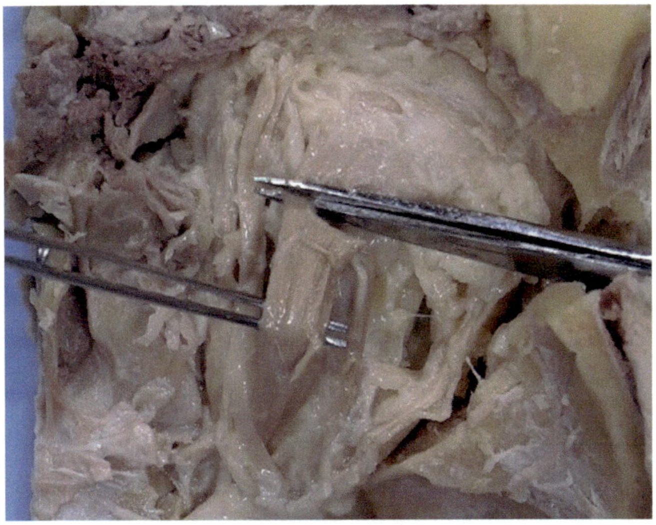

Fig. 5.22 The levator muscle, cut within the scissors

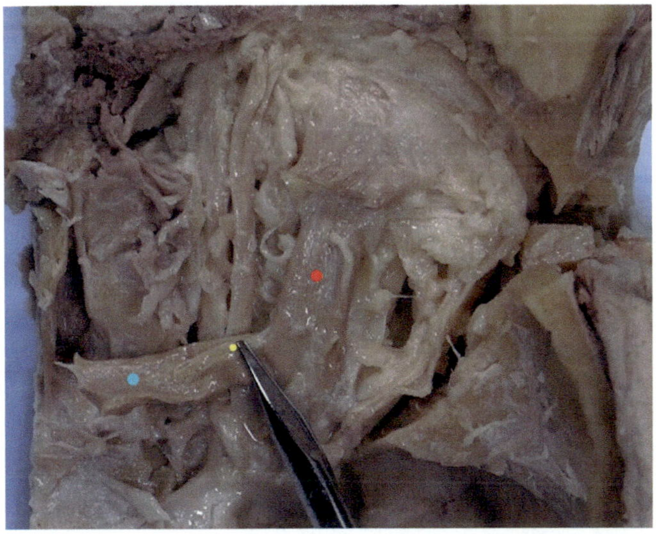

Fig. 5.23 The cut and reflected levator muscle (blue dot). The pointer is on the nerve (yellow dot) to the levator muscle. Note the superior rectus muscle (red dot)

Central Surgical Space (Muscle Cone)

10. Next, cut the superior rectus muscle 5 mm posterior to its insertion to the globe (Fig. 5.25), and reflect it, exposing the structures within the muscle cone. Now your removal of fat (Fig. 5.26) must be very gentle and careful.

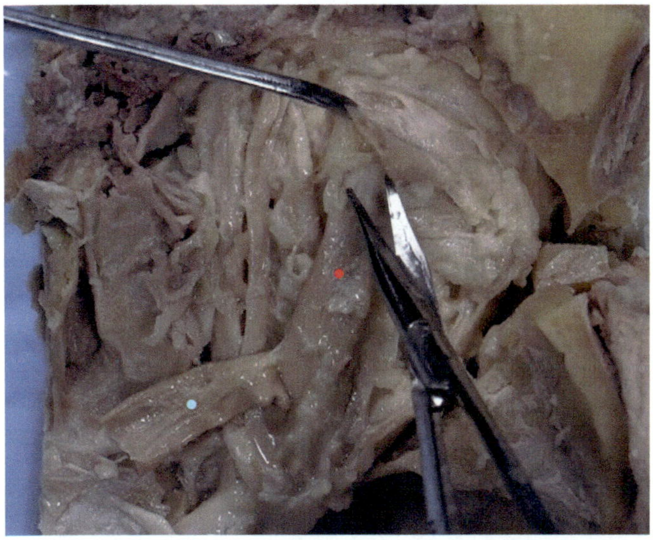

Fig. 5.24 Cutting fibrous attachments of superior rectus muscle (red dot) from the undersurface of the levator muscle stump (in forceps). Note the cut and reflected levator muscle (blue dot)

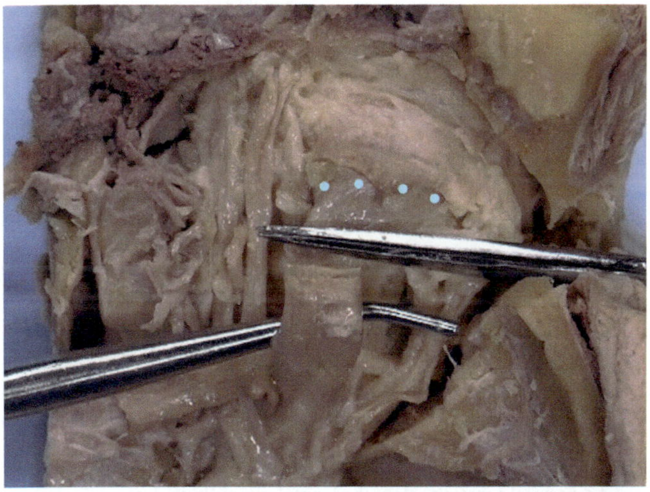

Fig. 5.25 The cut superior rectus muscle (above pointer) posterior to its insertion to the globe (blue dots)

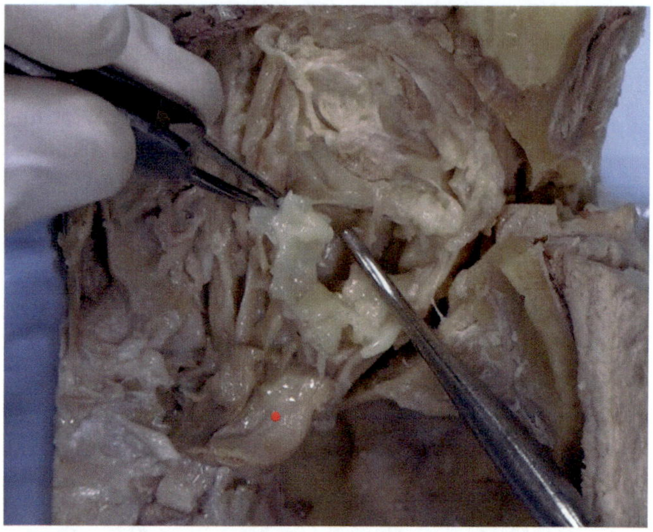

Fig. 5.26 Removal of intraconal fat (in forceps). Note the reflected superior rectus muscle (red dot)

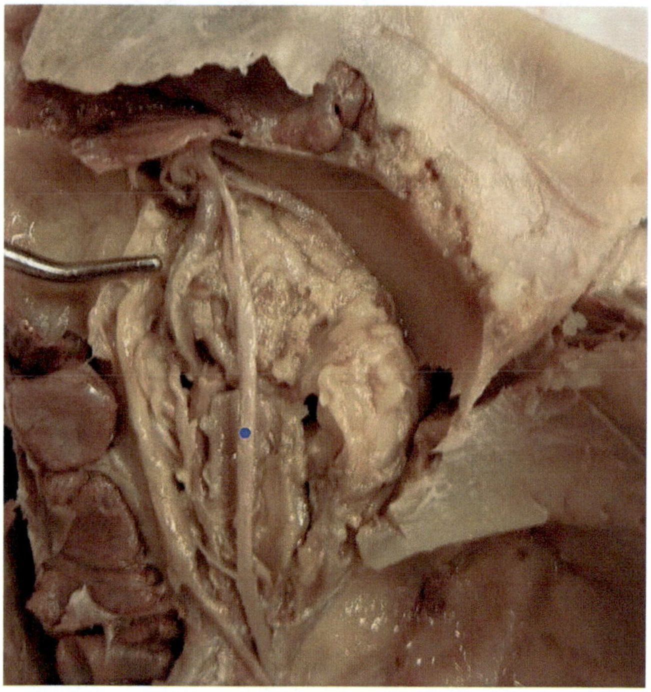

Fig. 5.27 The superior ophthalmic vein (pointer), in superior nasal anterior orbital location. Note the frontal nerve (blue dot)

11. Identify the *superior ophthalmic vein* passing from the medial and superior orbit (Fig. 5.27) to the lateral orbit into the muscle cone (Figs. 5.28 and 5.29).
12. Identify the *nasociliary nerve* (Fig. 5.30) and the *ophthalmic artery* (Fig. 5.31) crossing medially over the optic nerve.

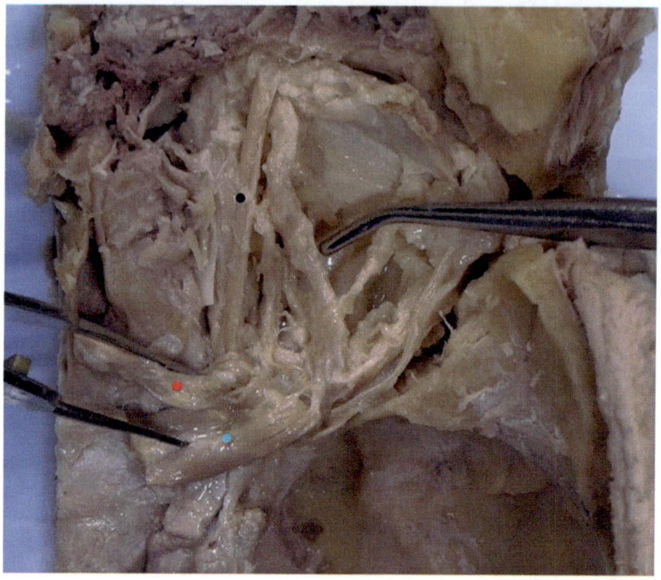

Fig. 5.28 The superior ophthalmic vein (pointer). Note the superior oblique muscle (black dot), the reflected superior rectus muscle (red dot), and the reflected levator muscle (blue dot)

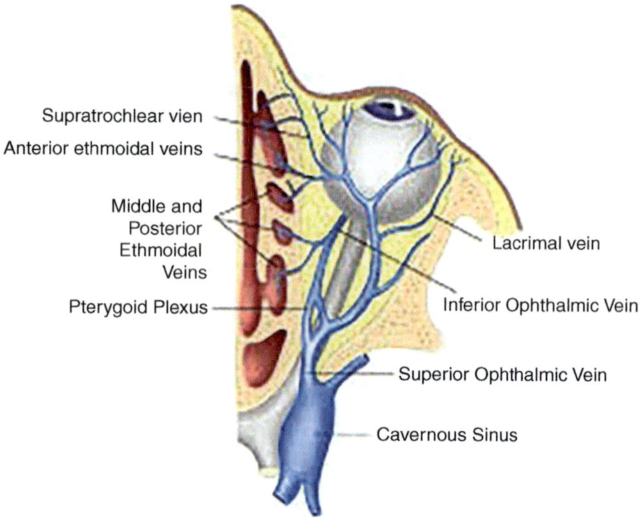

Fig. 5.29 Venous supply to the orbit

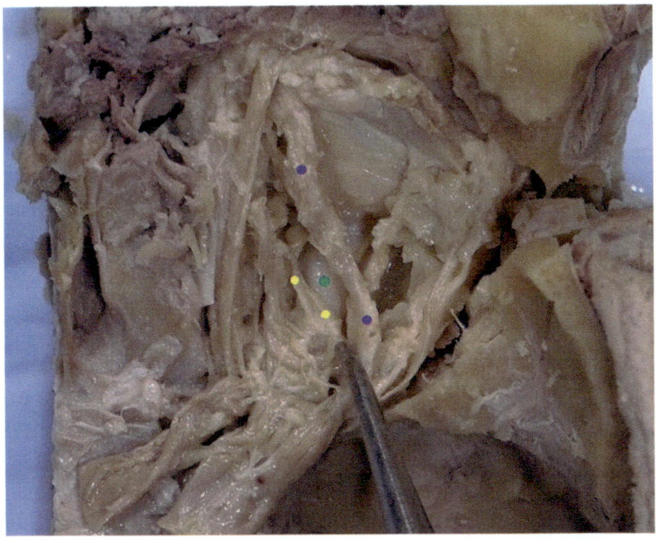

Fig. 5.30 The nasociliary nerve (pointer and yellow dots) crossing over the optic nerve (green dot). Note the superior ophthalmic vein (purple dots)

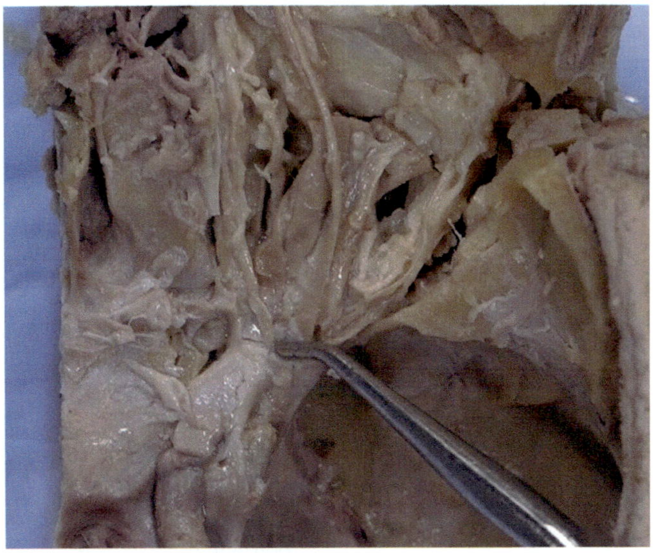

Fig. 5.32 The annulus of Zinn

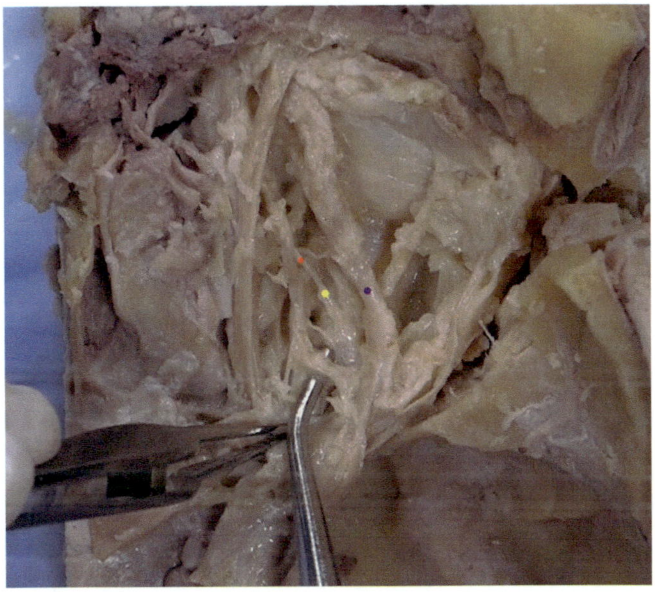

Fig. 5.31 The ophthalmic artery, on pointer. Note the nasociliary nerve (yellow dot), coursing anteriorly and nasally to become the infratrochlear nerve (orange dot). Note the superior ophthalmic vein (purple dot)

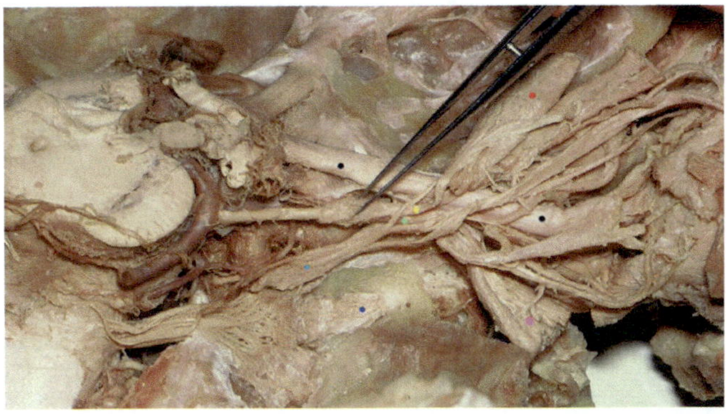

Fig. 5.33 The cavernous sinus and lateral view of the right orbit. The oculomotor (third) nerve (in forceps) is seen in the cavernous sinus where it divides before entering the orbit into the *superior division* (yellow dot) innervating the superior rectus muscle (red dot) and the *inferior division* (green dot) innervating the inferior rectus muscle (pink dot). Note the optic nerve (black dots), the ophthalmic nerve (light blue dot), and the infraorbital nerve (dark blue dot)

13. Clean the dura from the orbital apex to expose the annulus of Zinn (Fig. 5.32). Open the *annulus of Zinn.*
14. Trace the superior ramus of the oculomotor nerve posteriorly to find where it divides (Figs. 5.33 and 5.34) just before entering the orbit.

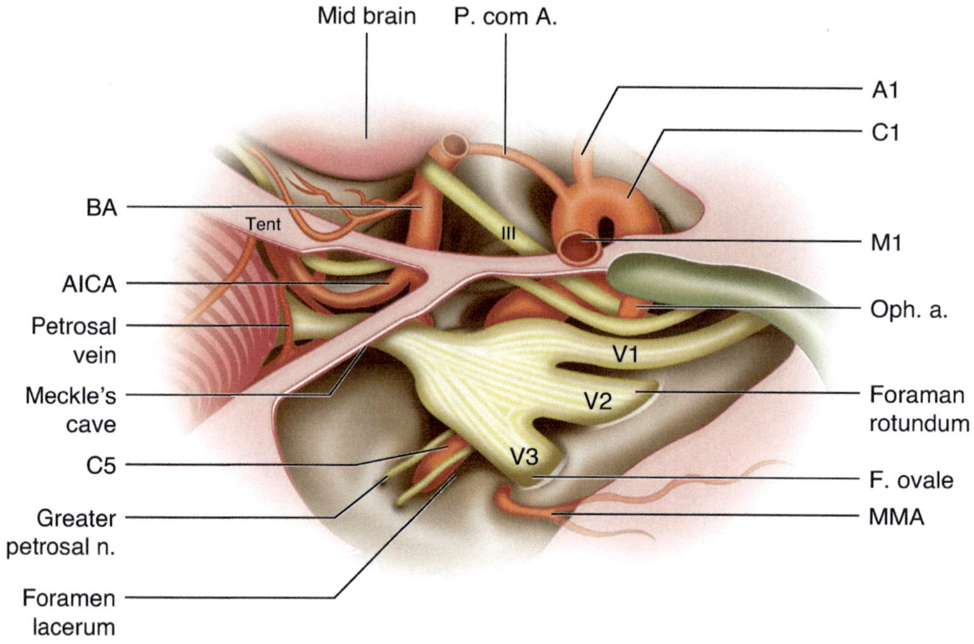

Fig. 5.34 Cavernous sinus

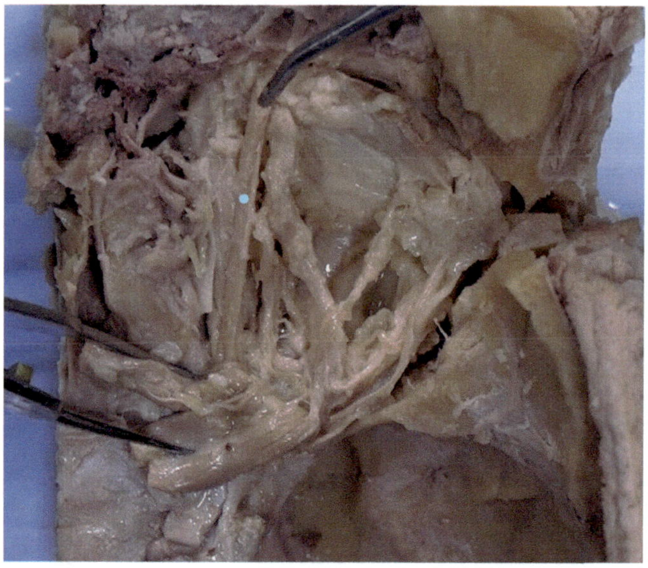

Fig. 5.35 The superior oblique muscle (blue dot). The anterior pointer is near the trochlea

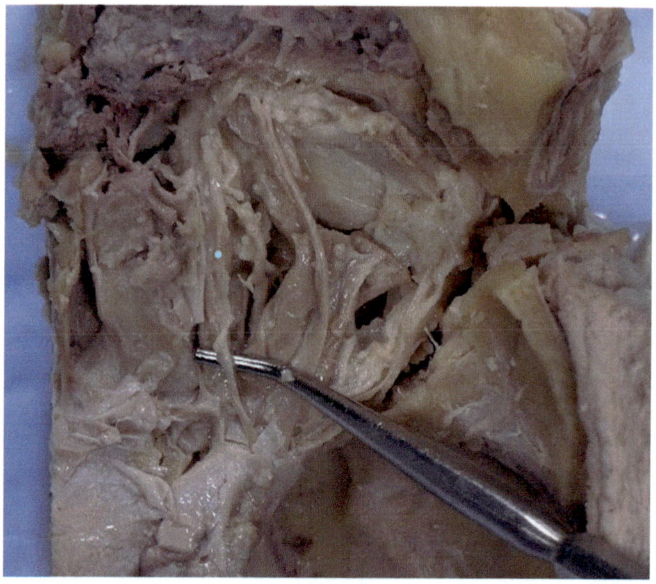

Fig. 5.36 The trochlear nerve (pointer) entering the posterior superior edge of the superior oblique muscle (blue dot)

15. Recall how the trochlear nerve lies on the lateral side of the cavernous sinus (*see* Fig. 4.12). Trace the superior oblique muscle (Fig. 5.35). Identify the trochlear nerve entering the posterior superior edge of the superior oblique muscle (Fig. 5.36).

Clinical correlation: From this viewpoint, it is clear why the superior oblique muscle, lying "outside" the annulus of Zinn, is not affected by a retrobulbar block.

16. Note the ophthalmic division of the trigeminal nerve entering the orbit as the lacrimal nerve (Fig. 5.37) and

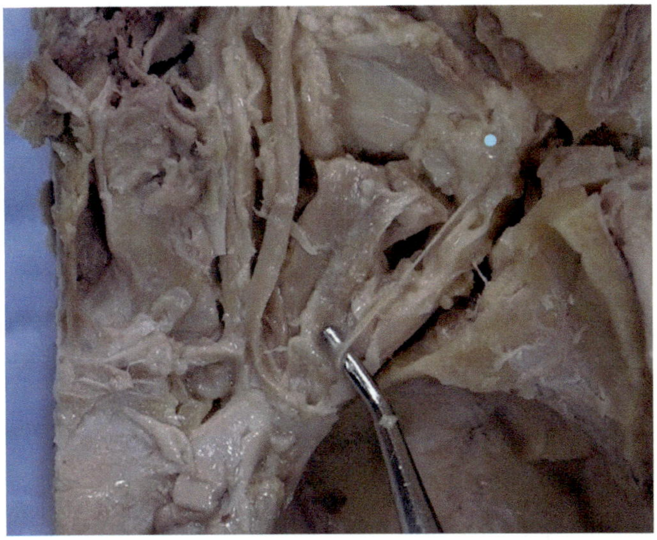

Fig. 5.37 The lacrimal nerve (on pointer) and orbital lobe of the lacrimal gland (blue dot)

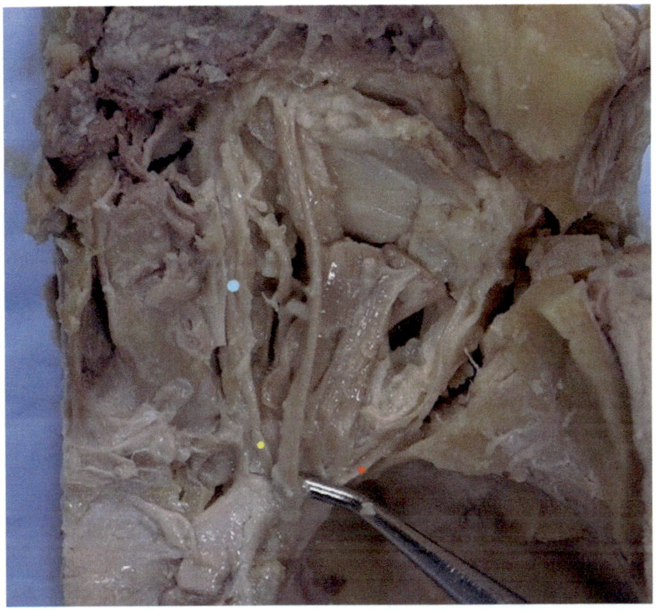

Fig. 5.38 The frontal nerve (pointer), superior oblique muscle (blue dot), trochlear nerve (yellow dot), and lacrimal nerve (orange dot), all outside the annulus of Zinn

the frontal nerve (Fig. 5.38) also above or "outside" the annulus of Zinn.

17. Trace the nasociliary nerve (Fig. 5.39) within the muscle cone as it passes nasally and anteriorly to become the *infra-trochlear nerve* (*see* Figs. 5.8 and 5.31).

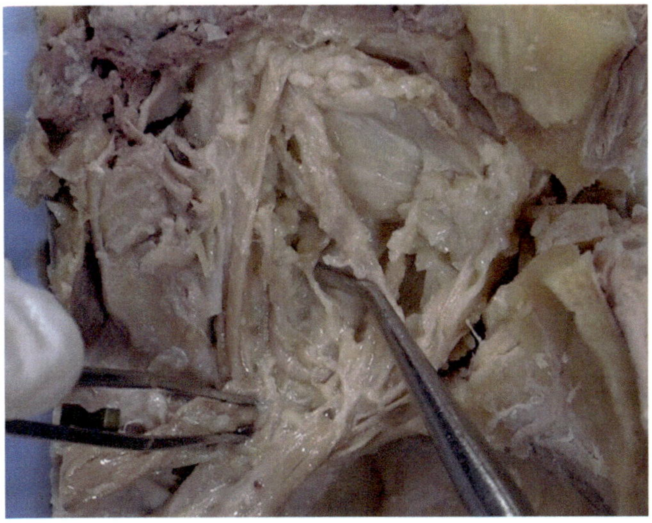

Fig. 5.39 The nasociliary nerve (pointer)

Clinical correlation:

1. It is easy to understand that the trochlear, frontal, and lacrimal nerves lie outside the muscle cone and are not affected with retro-bulbar blocks, but do affect the nasociliary nerve.
2. The ophthalmic artery (Fig. 5.31) is the only artery to supply the posterior orbit and, if occluded, will have devastating clinical effects.

Suggested Reading

Beard C, Quickert M. Anatomy of the orbit. 2nd ed. Birmingham, AL: Aesculapius Publishing Company; 1977. p. 23–34. 44-50

Della Rocca RC, Bedrossian EH, Arthurs BP. Ophthalmic plastic surgery: decision making and techniques. New York: McGraw Hill; 2002. p. 211–6. 222-4

Lemke B, Della Rocca RC. Surgery of the eyelids and orbit an anatomical approach. Norwalk, CT: Appleton and Lang; 1990. p. 36–9. 180-2

Whitnall SE. The levator palpebrae superioris muscle: the attachments and relations of its aponeurosis. Ophthalmoscope. 1914;12:258–63.

Zide M. Jelks G. Surgical anatomy of the orbit . Raven Press New York, 1985. pp. 51–57.

6 The Orbit: Lateral Approach

Edward H. Bedrossian, Jr

In this chapter, dissection of the orbit will continue from a lateral approach. First, the temporalis muscle will be removed exposing the temporal fossa. Next, the frontosphenoidal process of the zygoma and the bony lateral wall of the orbit will be removed exposing the lateral periorbita. Then, the lateral rectus muscle will be dissected, transected, and reflected, to enter the muscle cone. Next, structures within the muscle cone, including the ciliary ganglion, will be carefully dissected and identified. Clinical correlation will be provided.

Soft Tissue and Bone Removal

1. As seen in the shaded area of Fig. 6.1, the skin and temporalis muscle overlying the lateral frontal bone (Fig. 6.2), the zygomatic arch (Fig. 6.3), and the zygomatic process of the temporal bone (Fig. 6.4) are to be incised and elevated from the temporal fossa (Fig. 6.5).
2. Redirect your attention back to the orbit. Within the subperiorbital space, elevate the periorbita with its contained orbital structures from the lateral orbital wall and orbital floor.

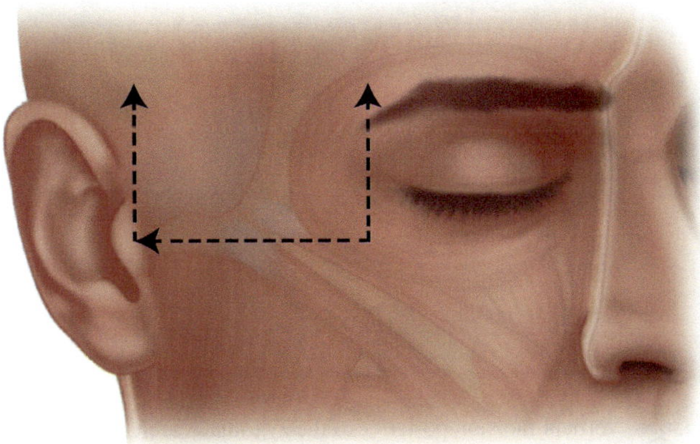

Fig. 6.1 Drawing of the skin and temporalis muscle to be excised

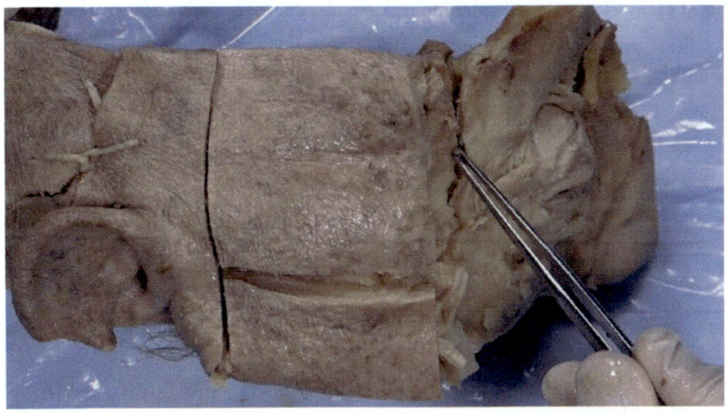

Fig. 6.2 Vertical incision posterior to the lateral orbital rim

E. H. Bedrossian, Jr, MD, FACS (✉)
Wills Eye Hospital, Philadelphia, PA, USA

E. H. Bedrossian, Jr et al. (eds.), *Anatomy of the Eyelid, Orbit, and Lacrimal System*,
https://doi.org/10.1007/978-3-030-88265-5_6

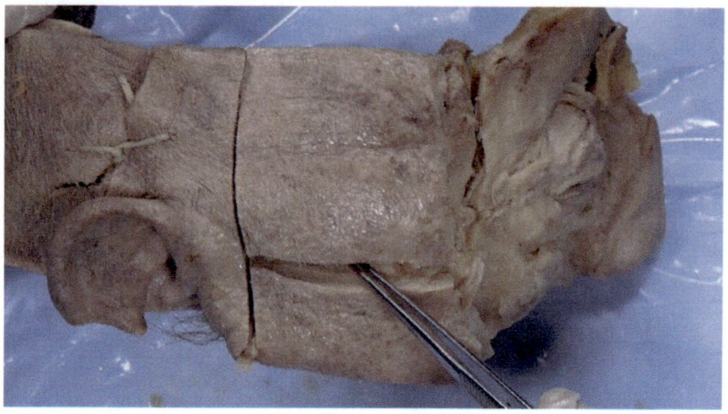

Fig. 6.3 Horizontal incision along the zygomatic arch

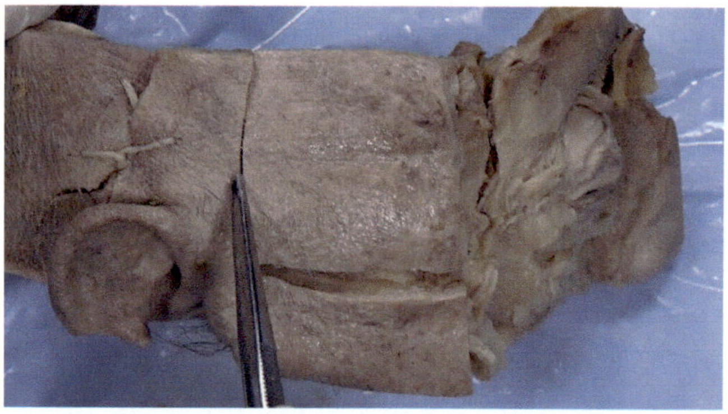

Fig. 6.4 Vertical incision posterior to the zygomatic arch

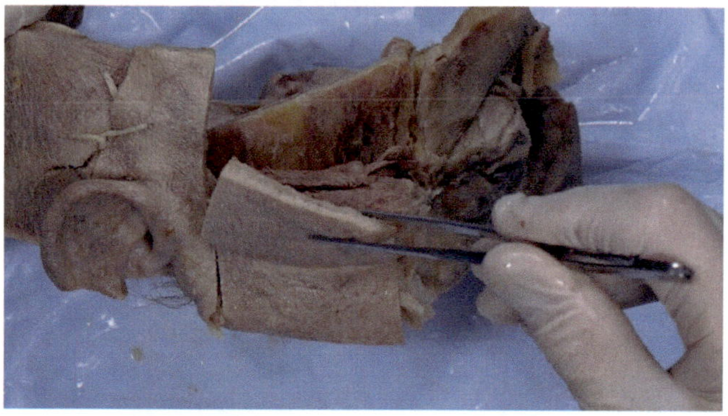

Fig. 6.5 Dissected skin and temporalis muscle removed exposing the temporal fossa

3. Using a saw or osteotome and mallet, cut vertically as shown in Fig. 6.1, through the lateral orbital wall (Figs. 6.6 and 6.7) and temporal bone (Figs. 6.8 and 6.9).
4. Remove the isolated bone (Fig. 6.10), separating the orbit (Fig. 6.11) from the middle cranial fossa (Fig. 6.12).

Clinical correlation: Knowledge of the dimension of the lateral orbital wall and its relationship to the middle cranial fossa are needed when performing lateral orbitotomy procedures.

5. Excise the exposed periorbita carefully.

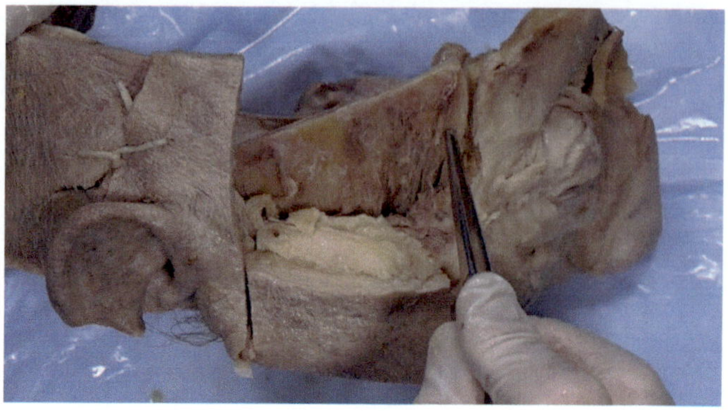

Fig. 6.6 Site for vertical bone cut through the lateral orbital wall (pointer)

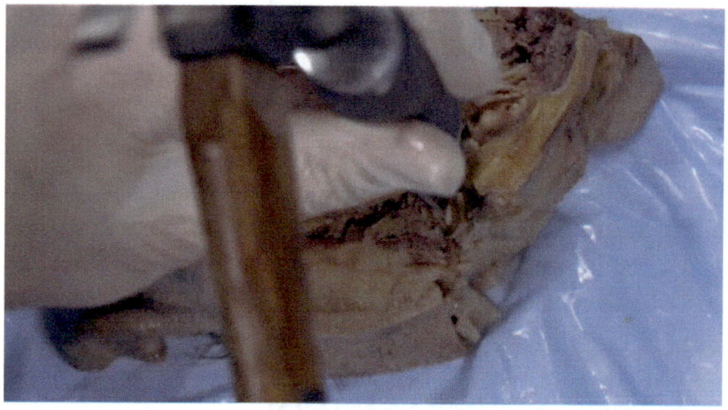

Fig. 6.7 Vertical cut with osteotome and mallet, through the lateral orbital wall

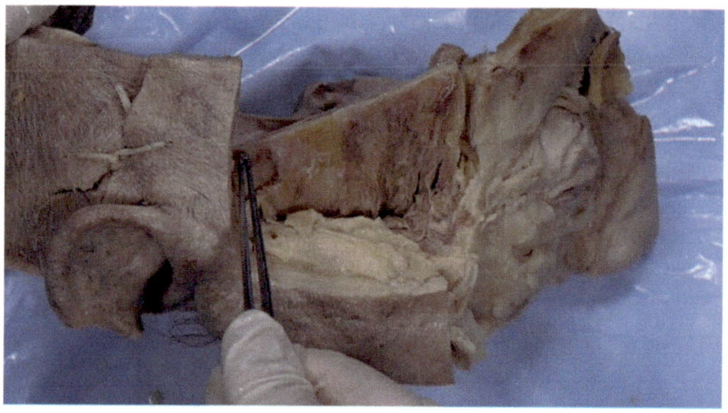

Fig. 6.8 Site of posterior cut through temporal bone (pointer)

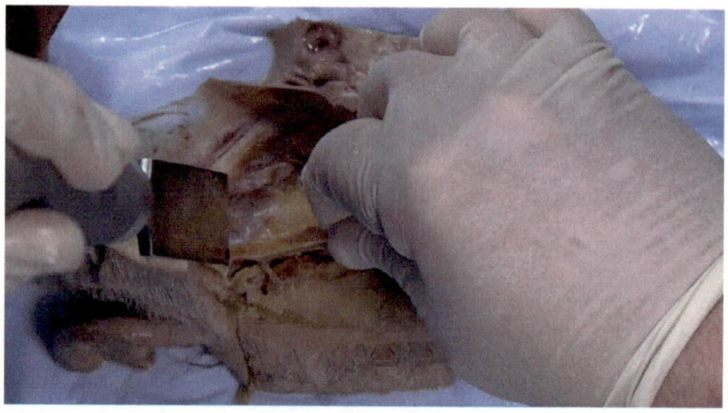

Fig. 6.9 Vertical cut with osteotome and mallet, through temporal bone

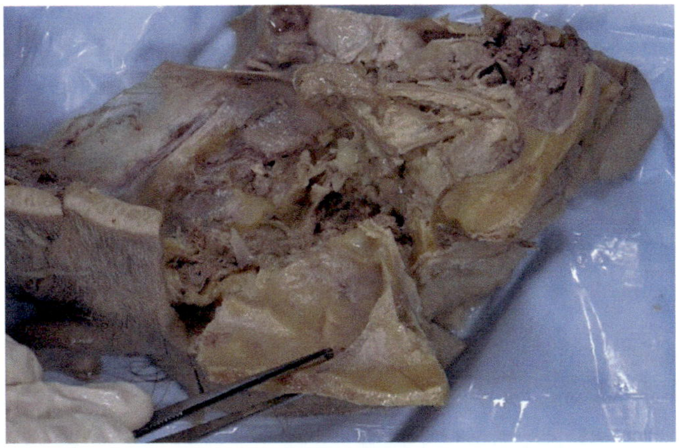

Fig. 6.10 Removal of the isolated temporal bone and greater wing of the sphenoid bone, separating the orbit from the middle cranial fossa

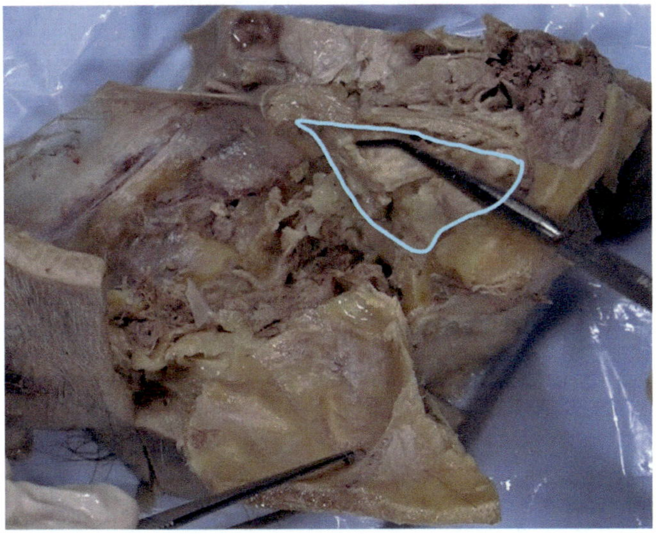

Fig. 6.11 Pointer resting on orbit, outlined in blue

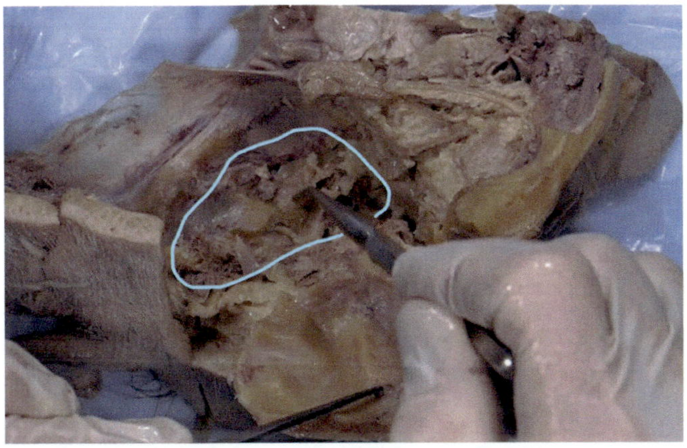

Fig. 6.12 Pointer over middle cranial fossa, outlined in blue

Lacrimal Gland

6. Dissect the lacrimal gland (Fig. 6.13) with the attendant artery, vein, and nerve (Fig. 6.14). Note how the gland is divided into a larger orbital and smaller palpebral lobe by the levator aponeurosis (Fig. 6.15).

Clinical correlation: Tissue taken from the anterior aspect of the orbital lobe of the lacrimal gland, at the time of incisional biopsy, will safely avoid injury to the attendant artery, vein, and nerve which are found posteriorly.

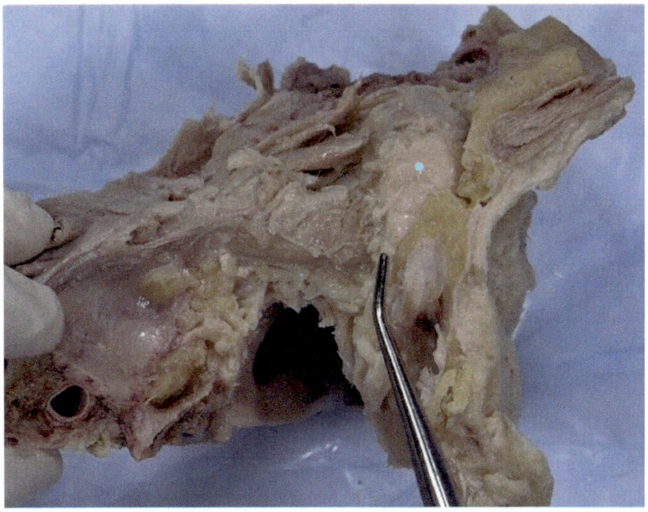

Fig. 6.13 Lacrimal gland (blue dot)

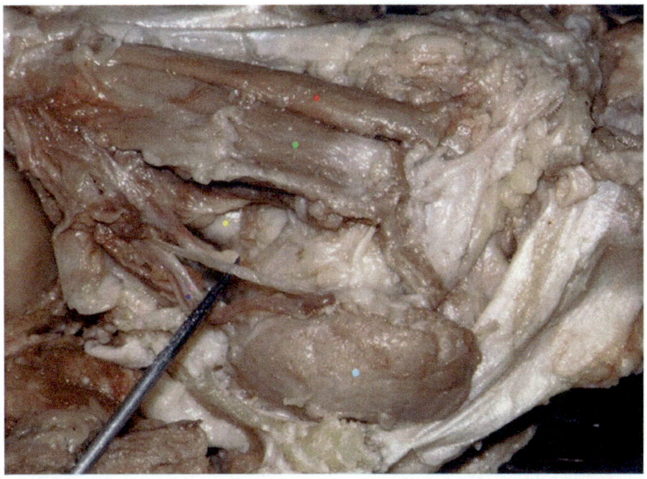

Fig. 6.14 Superior lateral view of the right orbit. Lacrimal nerve (pointer), lacrimal artery (pink dot), lacrimal vein (purple dot), lacrimal gland (blue dot), levator muscle (red dot), superior rectus muscle (green dot), and optic nerve (yellow dot)

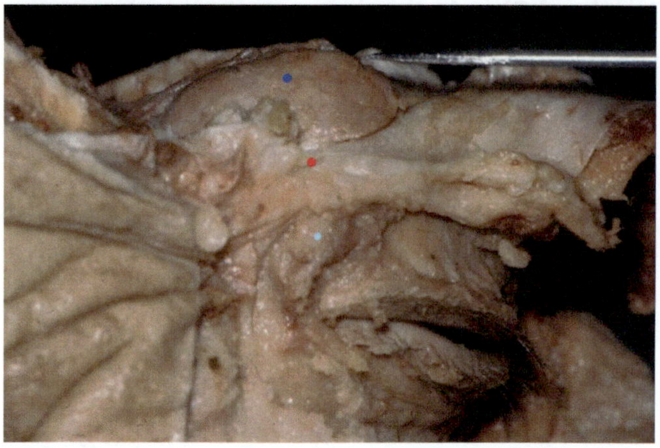

Fig. 6.15 The larger orbital lobe (dark blue dot) is separated from the smaller palpebral lobe (light blue dot) by the levator aponeurosis (red dot)

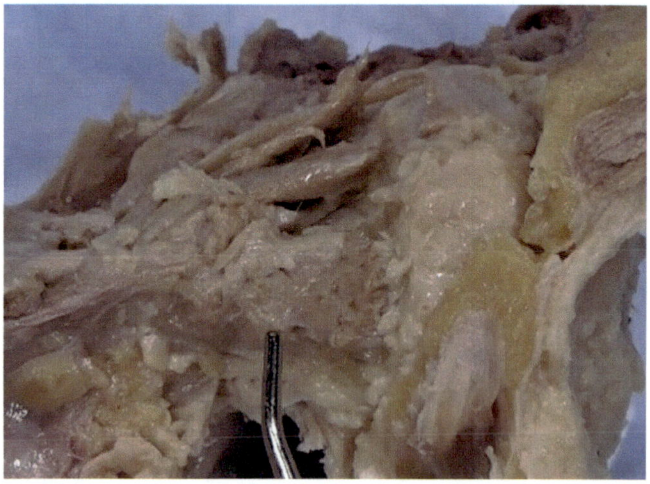

Fig. 6.16 Lateral rectus muscle

Lateral Rectus Muscle

7. Carefully clean the fat from above and below the lateral rectus muscle (Fig. 6.16).
8. Cut the lateral rectus muscle 5 mm posterior to its insertion onto the globe (Fig. 6.17), and reflect it posteriorly exposing the insertion of the abducens nerve (Fig. 6.18).
9. Trace the abducens nerve (CN VI) posteriorly within the annulus of Zinn.

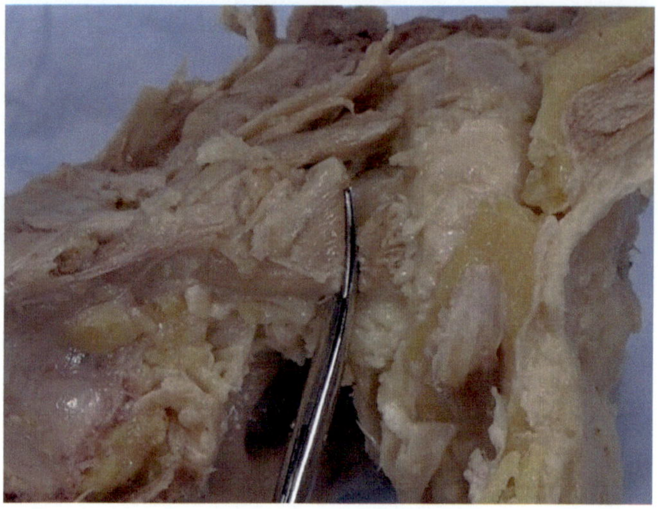

Fig. 6.17 Lateral rectus muscle cut, 5 mm posterior to its insertion

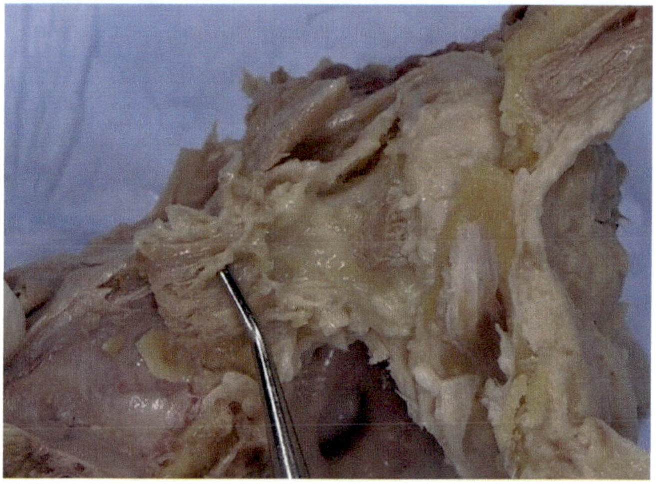

Fig. 6.18 Reflected lateral rectus muscle, exposing insertion of the abducens nerve

Clinical correlation: It is clear why retrobulbar blocks affect the lateral rectus muscle.

10. Identify and trace the superior ophthalmic vein (Fig. 6.19). Note how it courses from the anterior nasal orbit, crosses the optic nerve, and then is located posterior-lateral in the orbit.
11. Very carefully and gently clean the posterior globe and central surgical space of fat (Fig. 6.20).

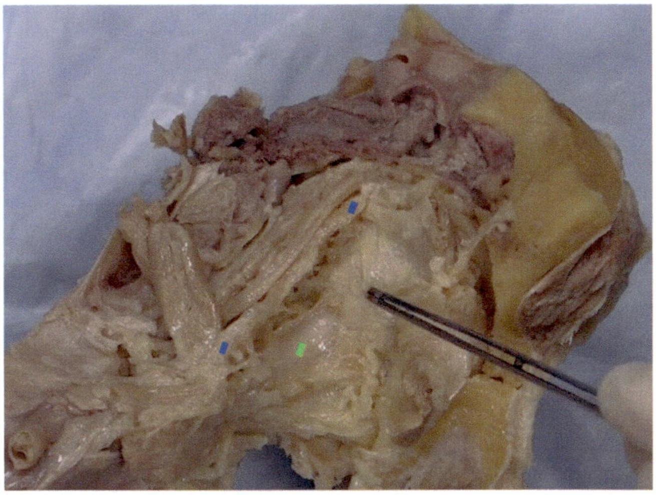

Fig. 6.19 Superior ophthalmic vein (between blue dots). The pointer is on the posterior sclera. Note the optic nerve (green dot)

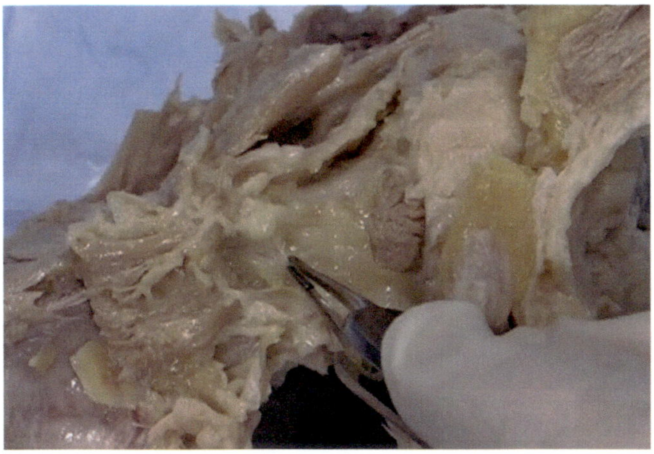

Fig. 6.20 Removal of fat within muscle cone with forceps

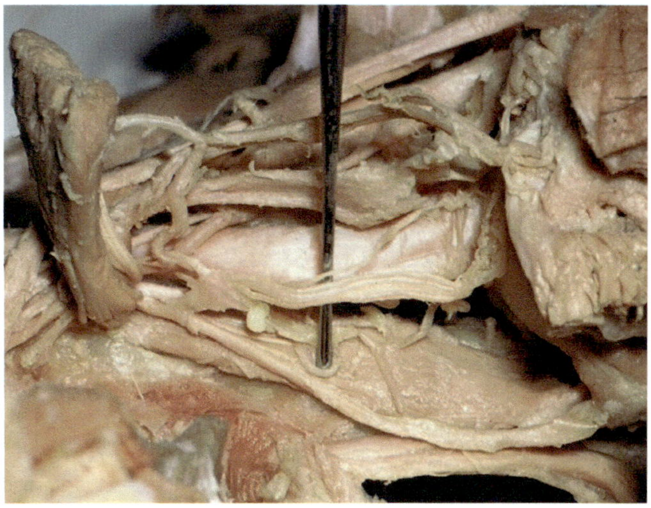

Fig. 6.21 The short posterior ciliary nerves elevated by the probe

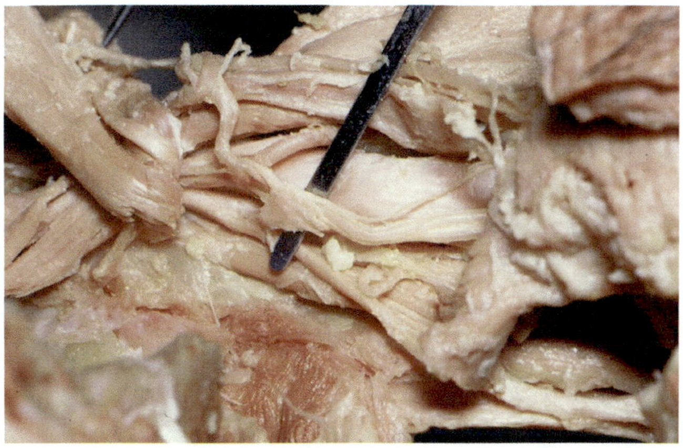

Fig. 6.22 The ciliary ganglion elevated by the probe

Ciliary Nerves

12. The short posterior ciliary nerves can be identified (Fig. 6.21). Trace these posteriorly to the small triangular ciliary ganglion (Figs. 6.22 and 6.23) located between the lateral rectus muscle and the optic nerve.
13. The nasociliary nerve is seen in the posterior orbit, lateral to the optic nerve, but crosses over the optic nerve (Fig. 6.24) to course medially anteriorly and superiorly

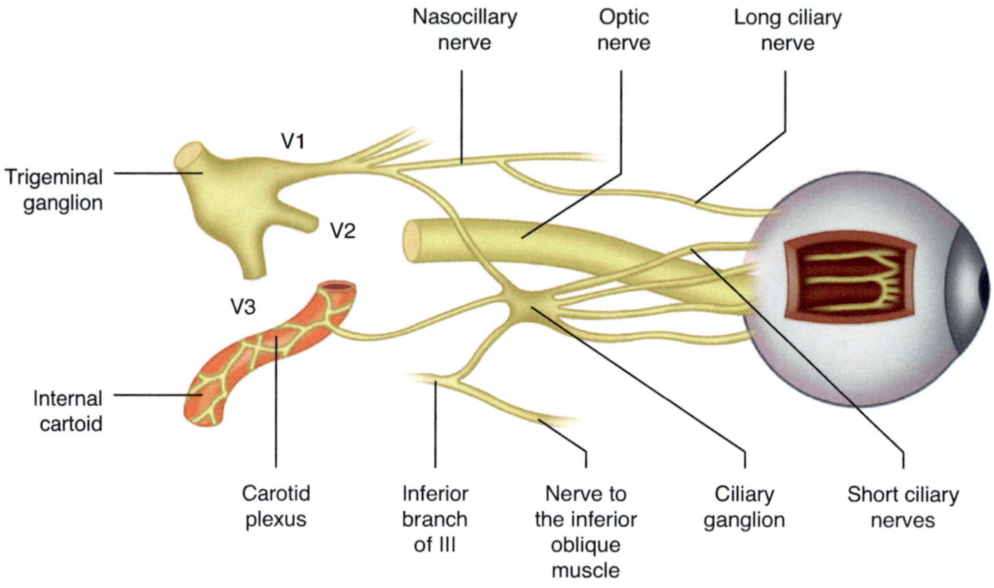

Fig. 6.23 Drawing of ciliary ganglion and it roots

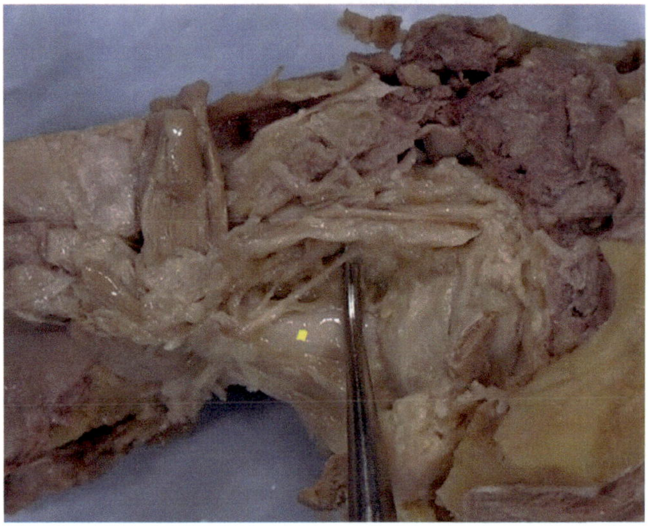

Fig. 6.24 The tip of the pointer is under the nasociliary nerve after it passes over the optic nerve (yellow dot). The nasociliary nerve then passes anteriorly under the trochlea to be renamed the infratrochlear nerve

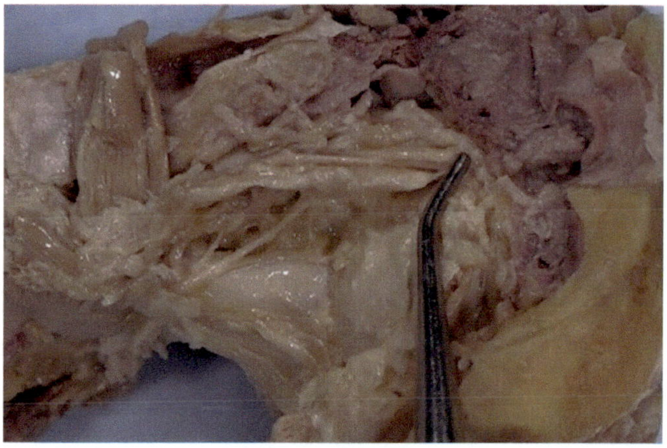

Fig. 6.25 Pointer on trochlea

in the orbit under the trochlea (Fig. 6.25) to become the infratrochlear nerve.

14. A sensory nerve connection is found between the nasociliary nerve and the ganglion (Figs. 6.26 and 6.27).

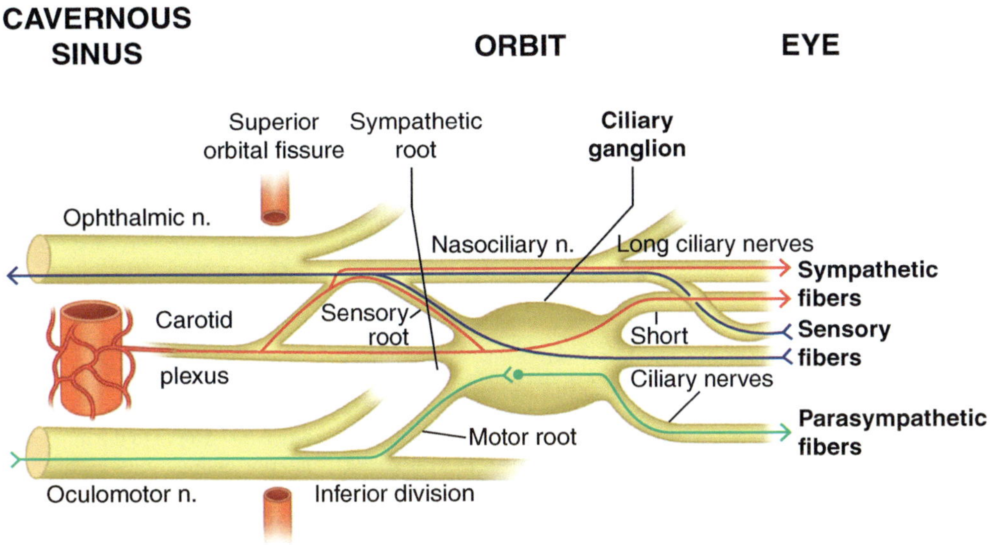

Fig. 6.26 Diagram of ciliary ganglion with the origin of its sensory, parasympathetic, and sympathetic fibers

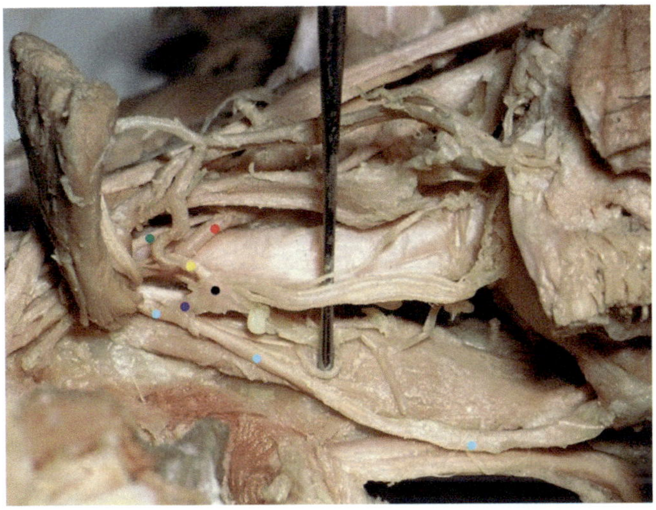

Fig. 6.27 Lateral view of the right orbit. Note the sensory nerve connection (yellow dot) from the nasociliary nerve, CN V1 (green dot), and the ciliary ganglion (black dot). Also note the parasympathetic branch (purple dot) from the nerve to the inferior oblique, CN III (blue dots), to the ciliary ganglion (black dot). The pointer is between the optic nerve and the posterior ciliary nerves. Note the ophthalmic artery (red dot)

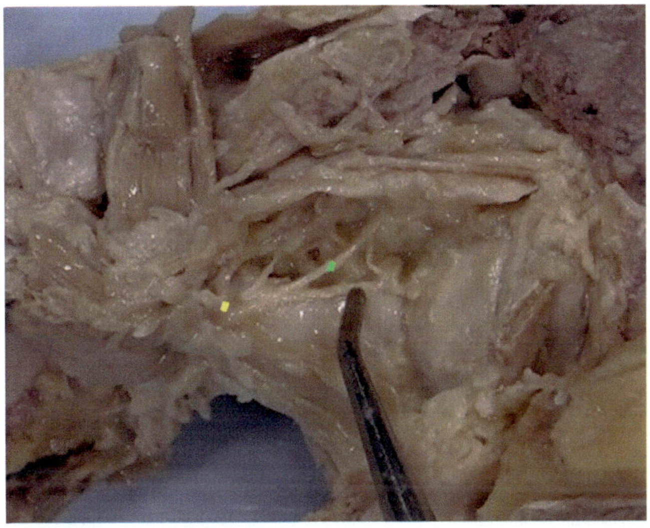

Fig. 6.28 Pointer on medial long ciliary nerve (yellow dot on ciliary ganglion; green dot on nasociliary nerve)

15. The lateral and medial long posterior ciliary nerves (Fig. 6.28) may be found running from the nasociliary nerve to the globe, without passing through the ciliary ganglion.

Clinical correlations:

(a) It is clear why retrobulbar blocks affect the nasociliary nerve to give anesthesia to the anterior segment.
(b) Extreme care is taken when operating in the lateral central surgical space to avoid injury to the ciliary ganglion and nerves.

Superior Oblique Muscle

16. Identify the insertion of the tendon of the superior oblique muscle (Fig. 6.29), and note its superior lateral relation to the globe and to the overlying superior rectus muscle.

Clinical correlation: Knowing this anatomy makes it easy to understand how the superior oblique depresses, incyclotorts, and abducts the eye. Therefore, a fourth nerve palsy will elevate, excyclotort, and adduct the eye.

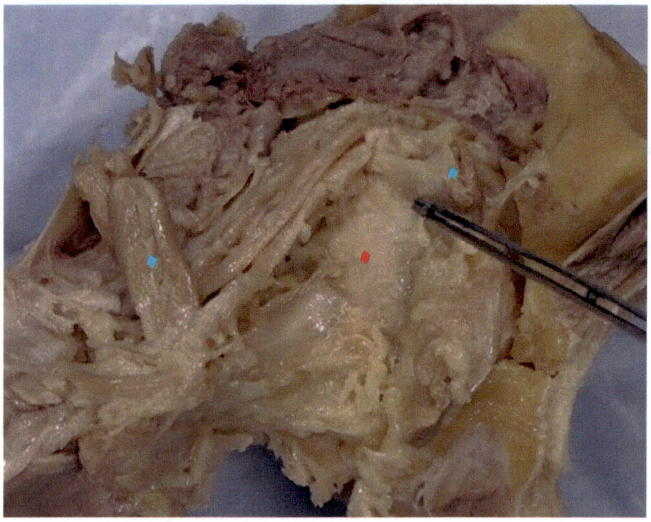

Fig. 6.29 Insertion of tendon of the superior oblique muscle in forceps. Blue dots on proximal and distal cut superior rectus muscle. Red dot is on the posterior sclera

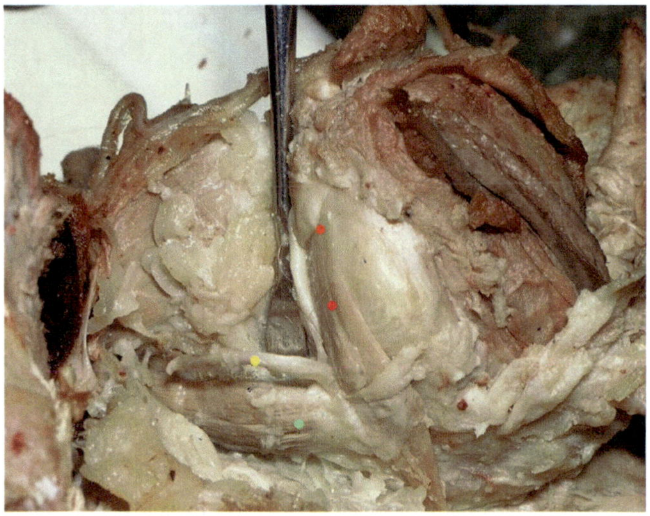

Fig. 6.30 Inferior lateral view of the right orbit. Note the inferior oblique muscle (red dot), inferior oblique tendon insertion (orange dot), inferior rectus muscle (green dot), and nerve to the inferior oblique muscle (yellow dot)

Inferior Oblique Muscle

17. Identify the fleshy insertion of the inferior oblique muscle (Fig. 6.30) inferolateral to the macula. It is the only extrinsic ocular muscle that does not arise from the orbital apex. It arises from the anteromedial aspect of the orbital floor, inferior to the bony lacrimal sac fossa. Note how the inferior oblique muscle courses beneath the inferior rectus muscle.

Clinical correlation: Knowing this anatomy makes it easy to understand how the inferior oblique elevates, excyclotorts, and abducts the eye. Therefore, a third nerve palsy involving the nerve to the inferior oblique will depress, incyclotort, and adduct the eye.

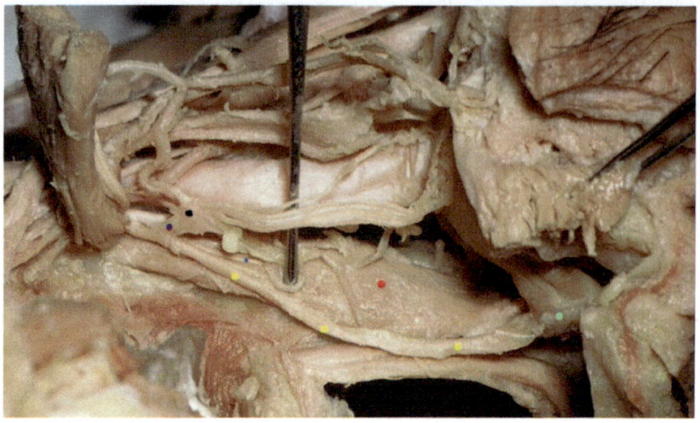

Fig. 6.31 Nerve to the inferior oblique muscle (yellow dots). Note the inferior oblique muscle (green dot), inferior rectus muscle (red dot), nerve to the inferior rectus muscle (blue dot), and parasympathetic nerve branch (purple dot) carrying parasympathetic fibers to the ciliary ganglion (black dot) from the nerve to the inferior oblique muscle. The pointer is between the optic nerve and the posterior ciliary nerves

18. Traveling along the lateral side of the inferior rectus muscle, identify the large nerve (Fig. 6.31) to the inferior oblique muscle. With further dissection, it may be possible to identify a vertical branch carrying pre-ganglionic parasympathetic fibers from the inferior oblique nerve to the ciliary ganglion (Fig. 6.26 and Fig. 6.31).
19. Identify the nerve to the inferior rectus muscle (Fig. 6.31).

Lateral Orbital Tubercle

20. The following structures have been disinserted from the lateral orbital tubercle of Whitnall and should now be identified:

- Lateral canthal tendon.
- Check ligament of lateral rectus muscle.
- Lacrimal fascia.
- Whitnall's superior orbital ligament.
- Lateral horn of levator.
- Lockwood's suspensory ligament.

Suggested Reading

Beard C, Quickert M. Anatomy of the orbit. 2nd ed. Birmingham, AL: Aesculapius Publishing Company; 1977. p. 34–43.
Della Rocca RC, Bedrossian EH, Arthurs BP. Ophthalmic plastic surgery: decision making and techniques. New York: McGraw Hill; 2002. p. 219–20.
Lemke B, Della Rocca RC. Surgery of the eyelids and orbit an anatomical approach. Norwalk, CT: Appleton and Lang; 1990. p. 289–95.
Lockwood CB. The anatomy of the muscles, ligaments and fascia of the orbit, including an account of the capsule of tenon, the check ligaments of the recti and suspensory ligament of the eye. J Anat Physiol. 1886;20:1–26.
Zide M, Jelks G. Surgical anatomy of the orbit. New York: Raven Press; 1985. p. 47–50,57.

Paranasal Sinuses and the Nasolacrimal Drainage System

7

Edward H. Bedrossian, Jr

In this chapter, the frontal, maxillary, sphenoid, and ethmoid sinuses will be examined first. Then the lacrimal sac and duct will be dissected. Clinical correlation is provided to stress the surgical and diagnostic importance of understanding the three-dimensional anatomic relationships of the orbit, the paranasal sinuses, and the nasolacrimal drainage system.

The Paranasal Sinuses

1. Examine the nose (Fig. 7.1). If your specimen has an intact nasal septum (Fig. 7.2), this needs to be removed (Fig. 7.3) to allow the study of the lateral nasal wall. The septum is a cartilaginous anterior extension of the vertical plate of the ethmoid bone.

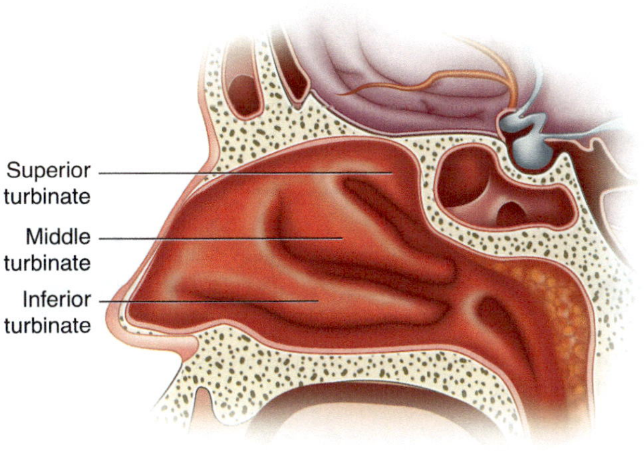

Fig. 7.1 Drawing of nasal passage. This medial view drawing of the lateral wall demonstrates the inferior, middle and superior turbinates

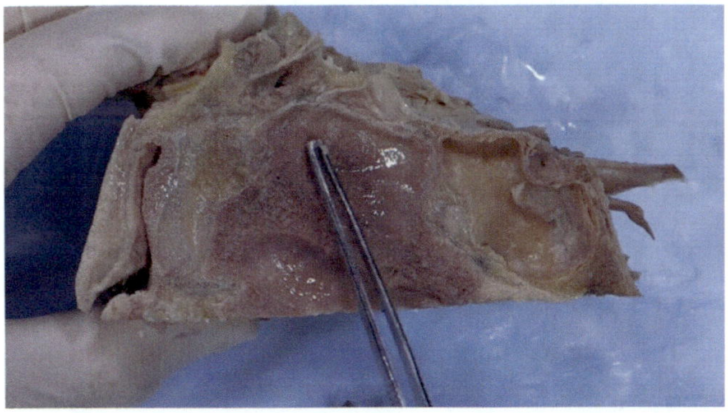

Fig. 7.2 Pointer on intact nasal septum

E. H. Bedrossian, Jr, MD, FACS (✉)
Wills Eye Hospital, Philadelphia, PA, USA

E. H. Bedrossian, Jr et al. (eds.), *Anatomy of the Eyelid, Orbit, and Lacrimal System*,
https://doi.org/10.1007/978-3-030-88265-5_7

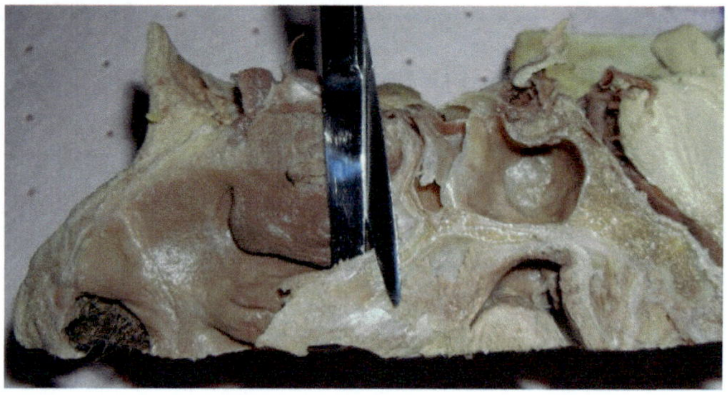

Fig. 7.3 Cutting nasal septum

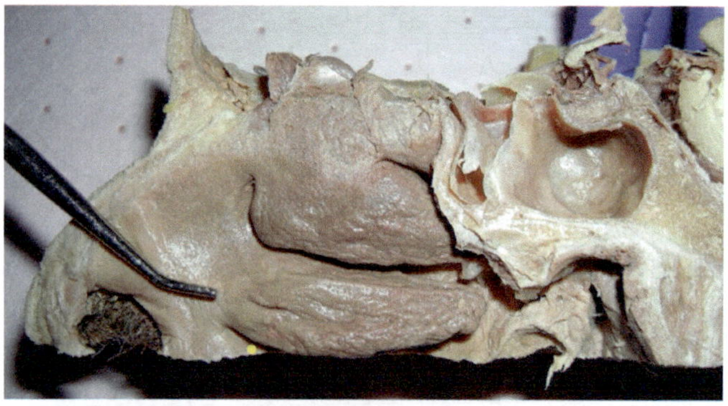

Fig. 7.4 Pointer on inferior turbinate. The inferior meatus is the space below the turbinate (yellow dot)

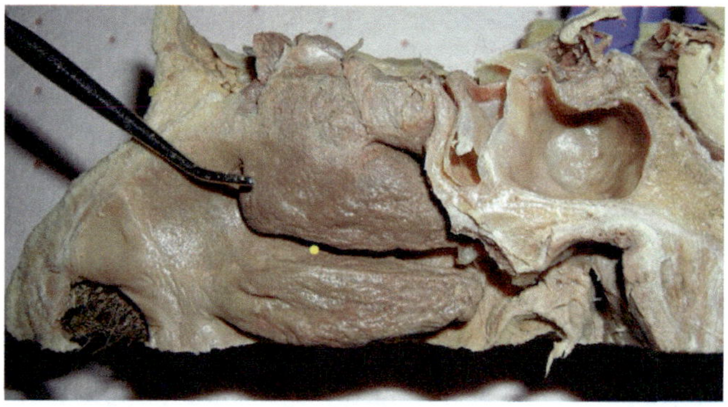

Fig. 7.5 Pointer on middle turbinate. The middle meatus is the space below the turbinate (yellow dot)

2. The inferior turbinate (Fig. 7.4), middle turbinate (Fig. 7.5), and superior turbinate (Fig. 7.6) can be seen arising from the lateral nasal wall. The space or "meatus" is named after the turbinate forming its roof. For example, the meatus between the nasal floor and the inferior turbinate is termed the "inferior" meatus. The turbinate bones are thin, almost completely pneumatized, and covered by nasal mucosa. The inferior turbinate comprises a bone unto itself and is seen attached to the medial wall of the maxillary sinus. The middle and superior turbinates are outcroppings of the ethmoid bone.

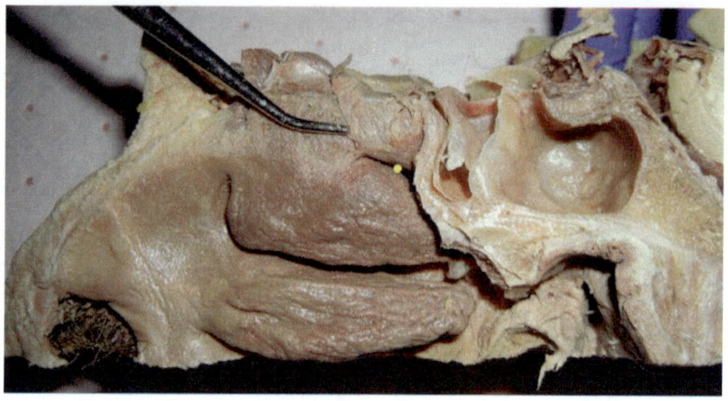

Fig. 7.6 Pointer on superior turbinate. The superior meatus is the space below the turbinate (yellow dot)

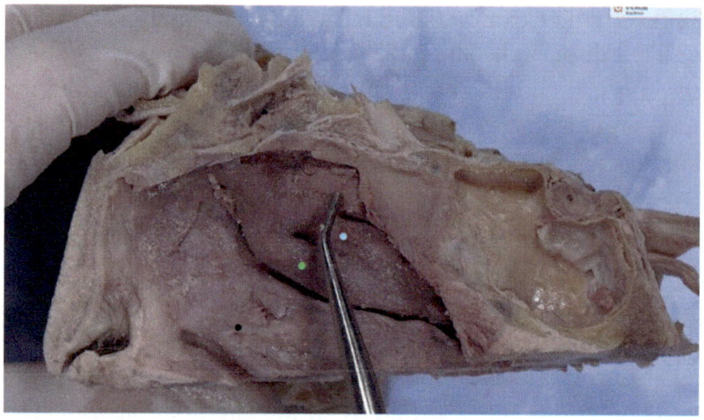

Fig. 7.7 Pointer on supreme turbinate. Note the inferior turbinate (black dot), the middle turbinate (green dot), and the superior turbinate (blue dot)

3. Occasionally, there may be a fourth or "supreme" turbinate (Fig. 7.7).

Clinical correlation: The natural tendency while examining the nose with a nasal speculum is to look superiorly into the middle meatus between the middle and inferior turbinates. However, with the patient in the examining chair, to examine the inferior meatus, a real effort must be made to gently rotate the speculum parallel to the floor, into an inferior anteroposterior axis (which may be uncomfortable).

4. Under the anterior portion of the inferior turbinate, approximately 3 cm posterior to the anterior nares, locate the valve of Hasner, which is the termination of the nasolacrimal duct (Figs. 7.8 and 7.9).

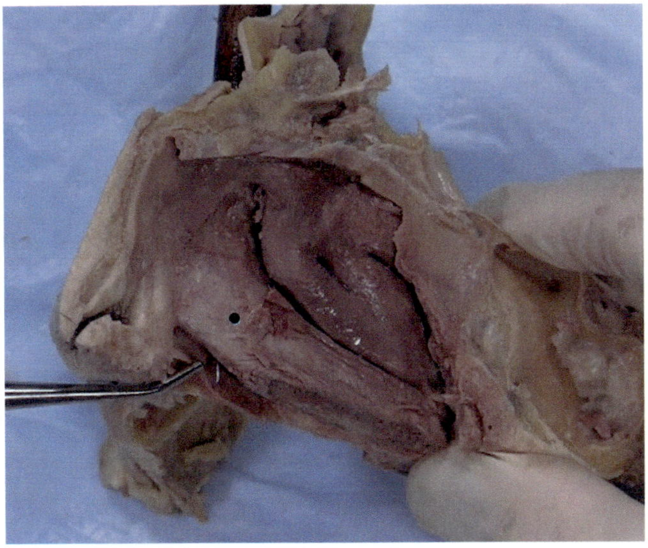

Fig. 7.8 Pointer under inferior turbinate (black dot), probe through the valve of Hasner at termination of nasolacrimal duct

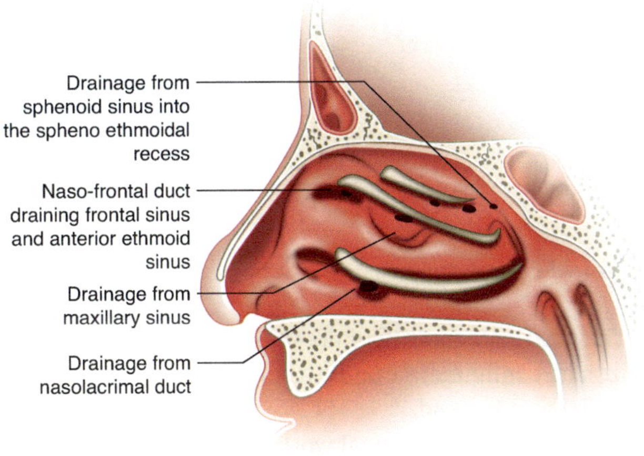

Fig. 7.9 Drawing of sinus drainage routes

5. In an analogous position underneath the middle turbinate, note the termination of the nasofrontal duct draining the frontal sinus and the anterior ethmoid cells (Fig. 7.9). The middle meatus, through separate ostium, also receives drainage from the maxillary sinus (Fig. 7.10) and the middle and posterior ethmoid cells.

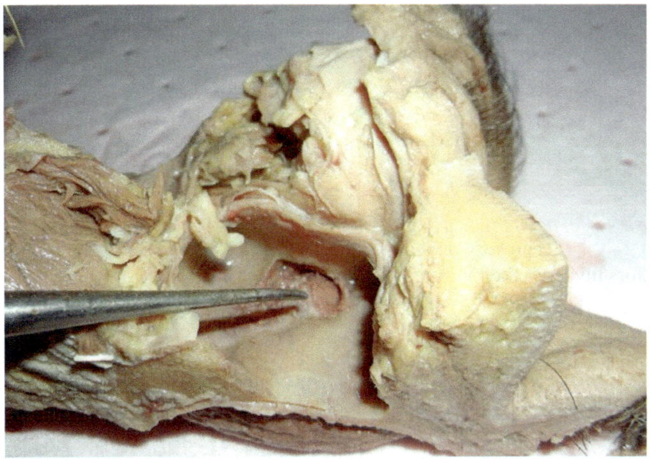

Fig. 7.10 Pointer on ostium in maxillary sinus. The lateral wall and floor of the maxillary sinus have been removed

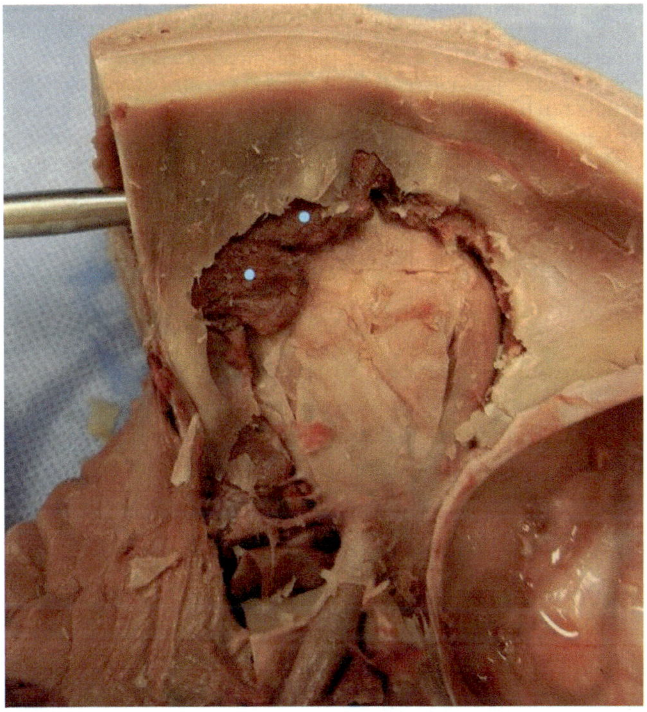

Fig. 7.11 Probe in large frontal sinus. Dots on frontal sinus mucosa

The Frontal Sinus

6. The frontal sinus (Fig. 7.11) may or may not be seen sectioned in your specimen. If so, attempt to locate the ostium draining the frontal sinus into the middle meatus (Fig. 7.12).

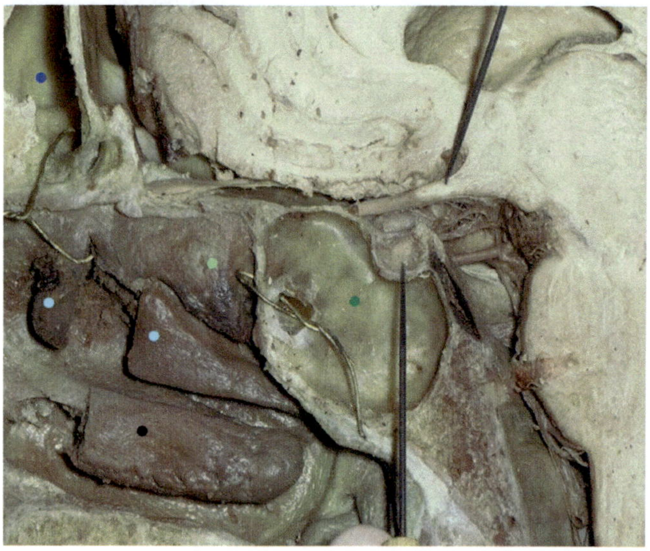

Fig. 7.12 The frontal and sphenoid sinuses. The upper left wire marks the ostium draining the frontal sinus (dark-blue dot) into the superior and anterior portion of the middle meatus. The middle turbinate (light-blue dots) has been partially removed exposing the middle meatus. The black dot is on the inferior turbinate. The center wire marks the ostium of the sphenoid sinus (dark-green dot) emptying into the superior-posterior portion of the nose under the superior turbinate (light-green dot). The optic chiasm is seen at the upper right pointer. The pituitary fossa is seen at the pointer from below

Clinical correlation: Evagination pits of the frontal recess (anterosuperior middle meatus) can be seen at birth, signifying the beginning of frontal sinus development, but X-ray evidence is not seen until age 6.

The Maxillary Sinus

7. Turn your attention to the maxillary sinus. Note the thin mucoperiosteum (Fig. 7.13) which lines this sinus and all the sinuses.
   Clinical correlation:

(a) Note the ostium high on the medial wall which is the site of the embryologic evagination from the nasal cavity.
(b) Functionally, the mucoperiosteum hosts cilia which in an organized fashion wave the mucous and foreign particles toward the ostium.

8. The roots of the upper teeth stand in relief on the floor of the maxillary sinus, but may or may not be seen in your specimen, as prepared.

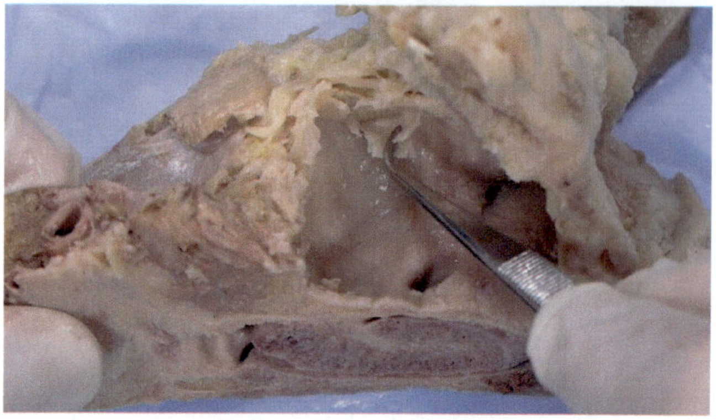

Fig. 7.13 Removal of mucoperiosteum of maxillary sinus

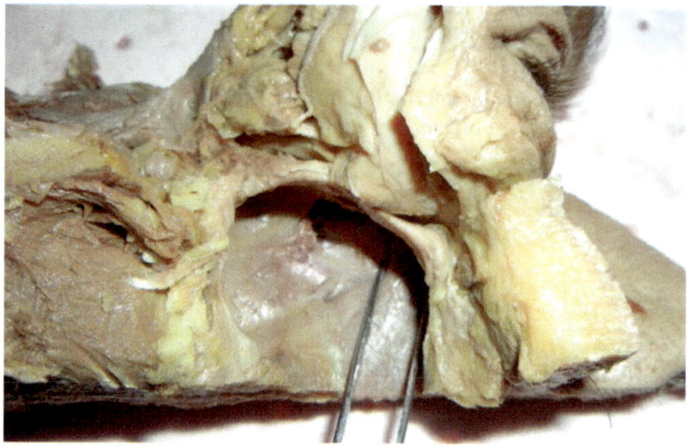

Fig. 7.14 Bony nasolacrimal canal within forceps

Clinical correlation:

(a) The maxillary sinus floor does not achieve the adult horizontal configuration until age 12 when all permanent teeth have descended.
(b) Infection following dental work on the upper teeth rarely can cause maxillary sinusitis and secondary orbital cellulitis.

9. Note that the bony nasolacrimal canal is a localized posterior, inferior, and lateral dilation of the medial wall of this sinus (Fig. 7.14).

The Ethmoid Sinus

The ethmoid bone should be considered as a box with multiple contained bullae (Fig. 7.15) as variable as the fingerprint. Only the outer lateral ethmoid walls (orbital) are constant.

10. Within the superior meatus, between the middle and superior turbinates (Fig. 7.6), strip away the nasal mucosa, and

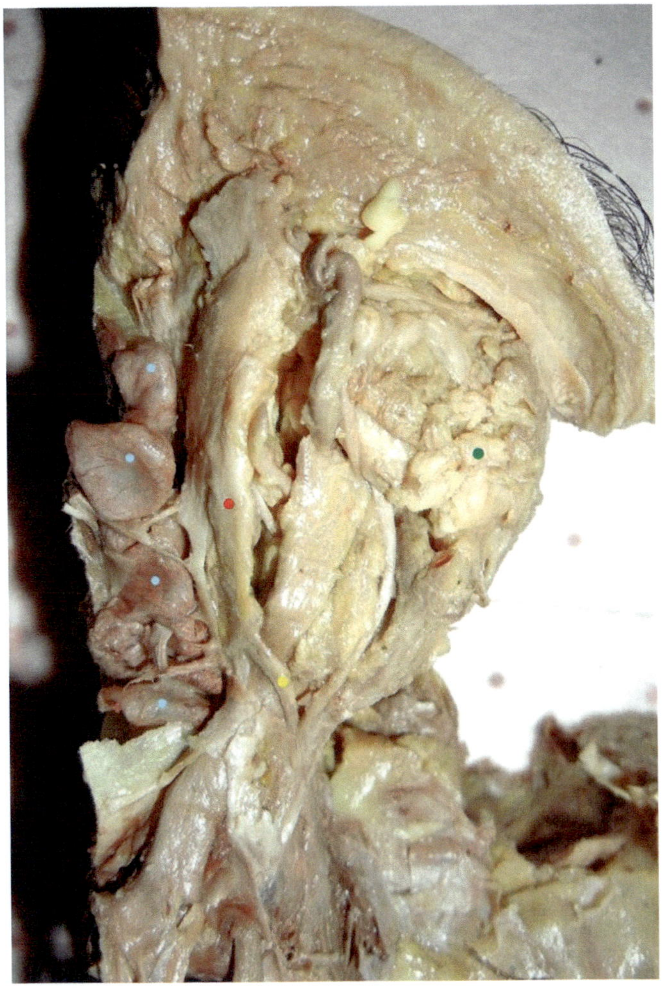

Fig. 7.15 Right ethmoid sinuses and orbit from above. Blue dots on ethmoid bullae, red dot on superior oblique muscle, yellow dot on trochlear nerve, and green dot on lacrimal gland

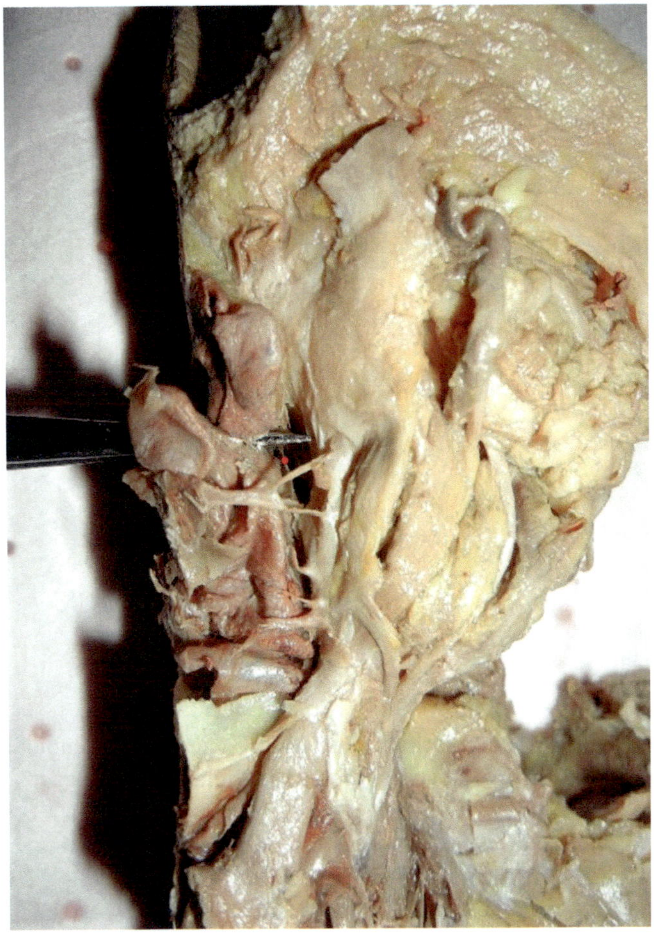

Fig. 7.16 Right ethmoid sinuses and orbit. Probe extending from superior meatus into the ethmoid sinus, perforating the thin medial orbital wall (red dot) into the orbit

then with a probe, break into the ethmoid sinus, pushing laterally until the medial orbital wall is perforated (Fig. 7.16).

Clinical correlation: The thin lamina papyracea of the ethmoid bone predisposes it to surgical and blunt trauma, as well as easy access for infectious and malignant processes.

The Sphenoid Sinus

11. The sphenoid sinus (Figs. 7.12 and 7.17) can be seen emptying into the most superior-posterior portion of the nose at the sphenoethmoidal recess, within the superior meatus. The sphenoid sinus represents the pneumatization of the body of the sphenoid bone and occasionally may extend into the sphenoid wings.

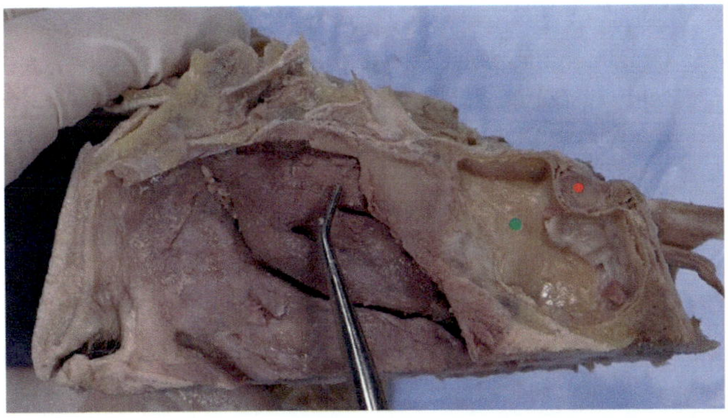

Fig. 7.17 Sphenoid sinus (green dot), pituitary gland/fossa (red dot). Pointer on supreme turbinate near sphenoethmoidal recess

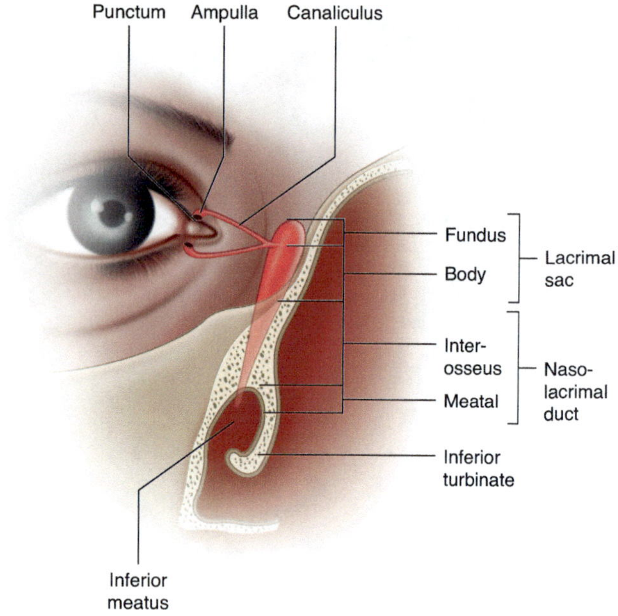

Fig. 7.18 Drawing of the excretory nasolacrimal system

Clinical correlation: The endoscopic transsphenoidal approach is used to access the pituitary gland.

The Nasolacrimal Drainage System

12. The nasolacrimal duct (Fig. 7.18) can be seen as a posterior, inferior, and laterally directed elevation of the medial maxillary sinus wall (Fig. 7.14). Remove the mucosa over the course of the nasolacrimal duct (Fig. 7.19), and piecemeal remove the maxillary bone exposing the membranous duct (Fig. 7.20).

13. Create an incision down to the bone of the anterior lacrimal crest (Fig. 7.21), and continue it up 1 cm above the medial canthal tendon.

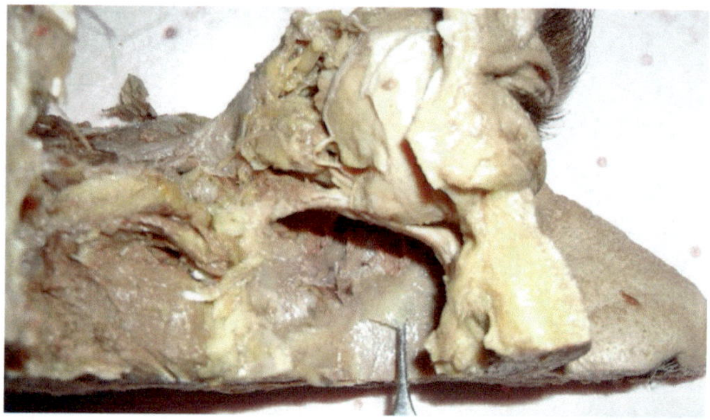

Fig. 7.19 Removal of the maxillary sinus mucosa over the course of the nasolacrimal duct

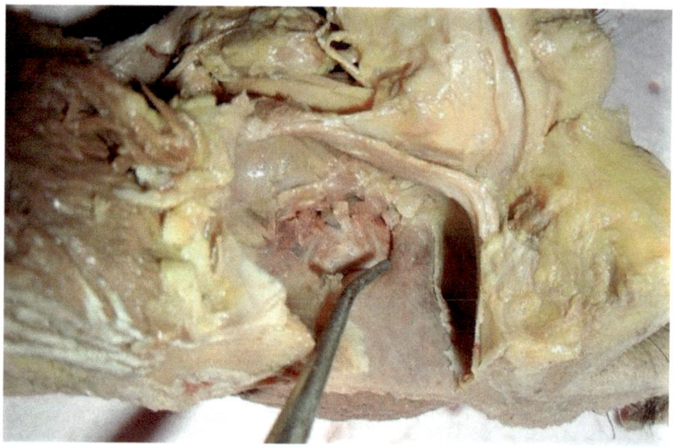

Fig. 7.20 Partially removed maxillary bone exposing membranous nasolacrimal duct

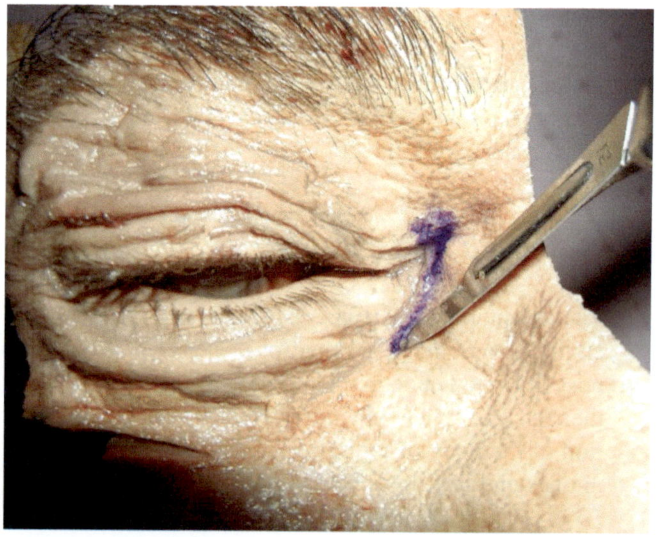

Fig. 7.21 Site of skin incision to expose the anterior lacrimal crest

14. Subperiosteally elevate all soft tissue laterally (Figs. 7.22 and 7.23) from the nasolacrimal fossa.
15. Using the exposed nasolacrimal duct as a starting point, dissect the anterior aspect of the lacrimal sac free of the encasing orbicularis muscle (Figs. 7.24 and 7.25). Soft tissue removal must be liberal.

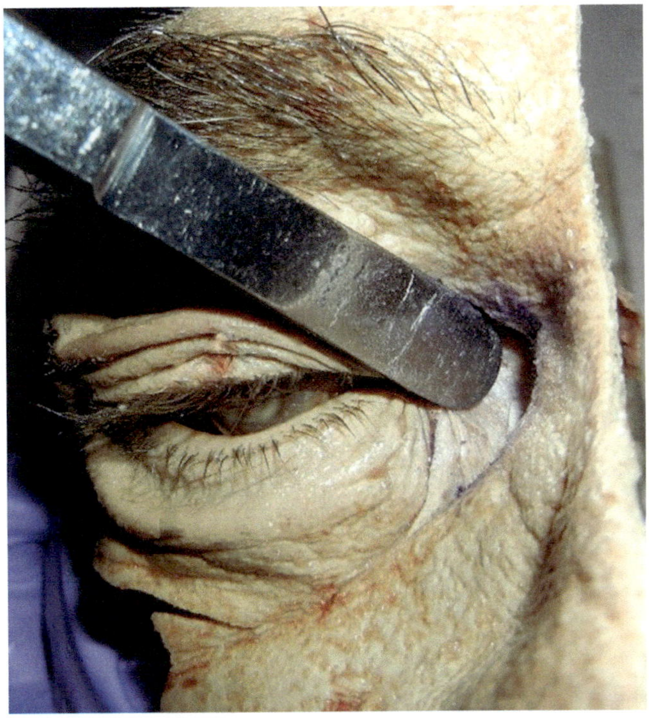

Fig. 7.22 Elevation of soft tissue laterally to expose anterior lacrimal crest

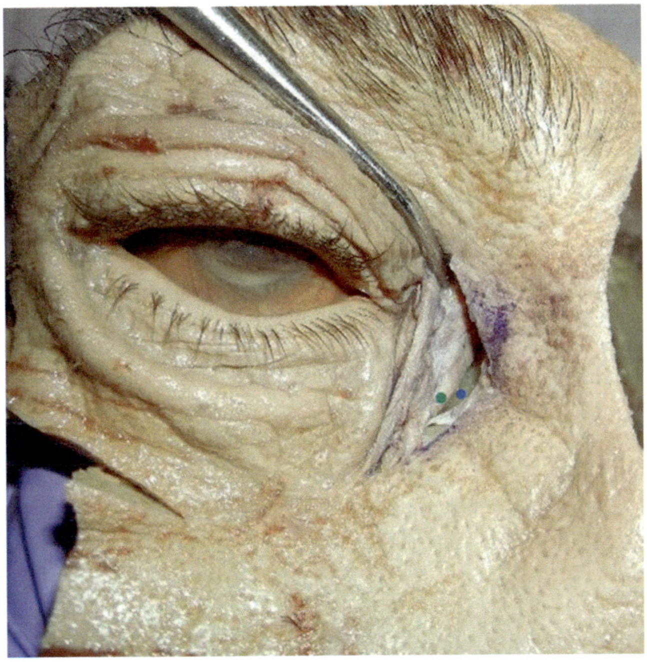

Fig. 7.23 Subperiosteal incision exposing anterior lacrimal crest (blue dot). Pointer is retracting skin, exposing lacrimal sac (green dot)

16. Further removal of the anterior lacrimal crest and bony canal will expose the entire membranous nasolacrimal system (Fig. 7.26).

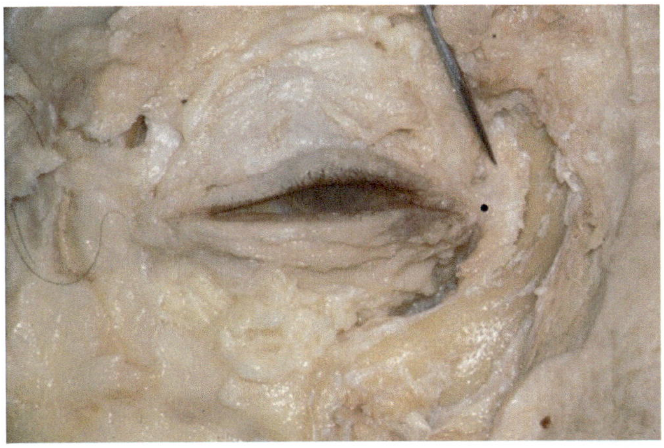

Fig. 7.24 Fundus of the lacrimal sac above medial canthal tendon (black dot)

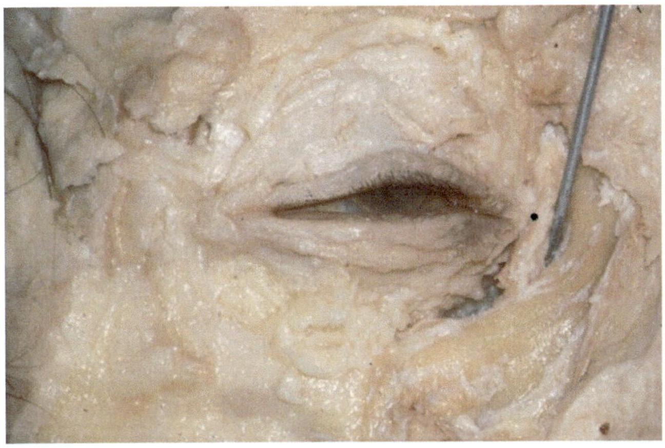

Fig. 7.25 Body of the lacrimal sac below medial canthal tendon (black dot)

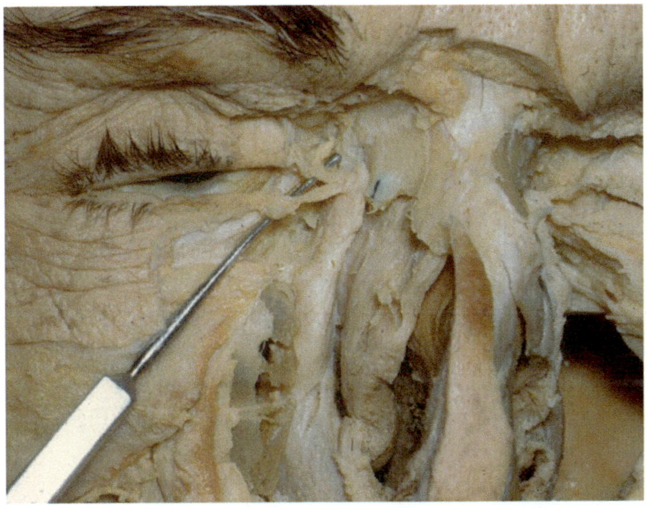

Fig. 7.26 Soft tissue and bone removed, exposing membranous nasolacrimal drainage system. Pointer is under the superior and inferior canaliculi

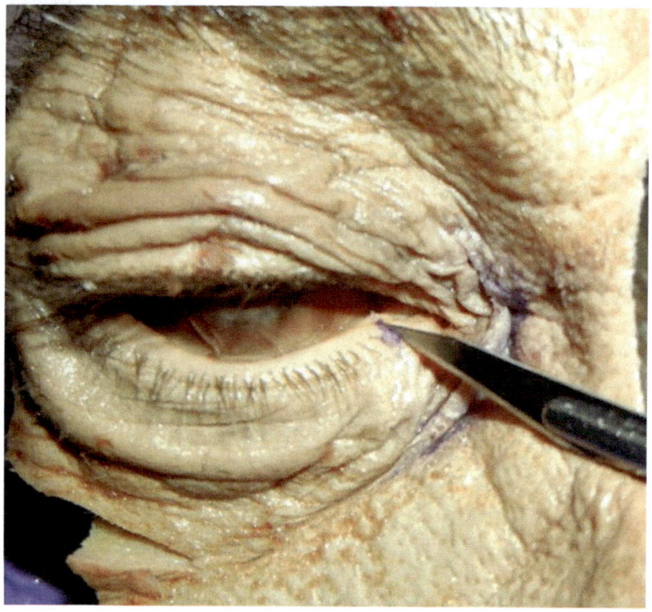

Fig. 7.27 Vertical incision at the punctum

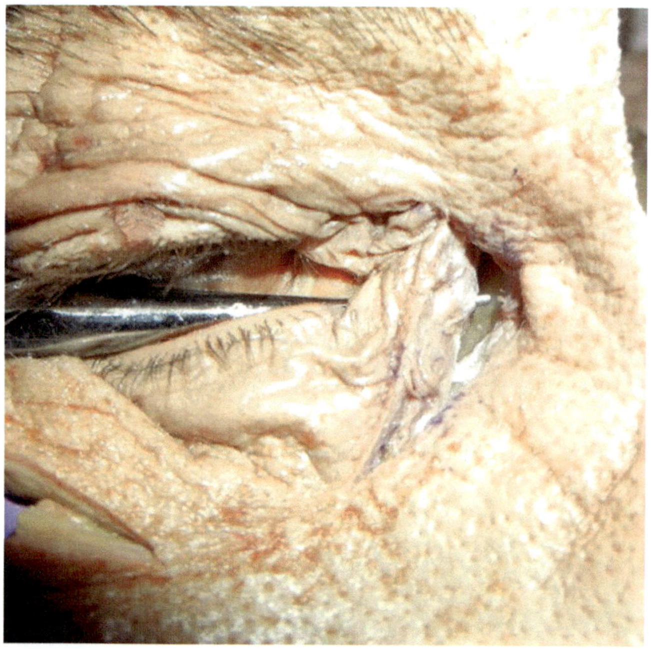

Fig. 7.28 Probe through the canaliculus into the sac

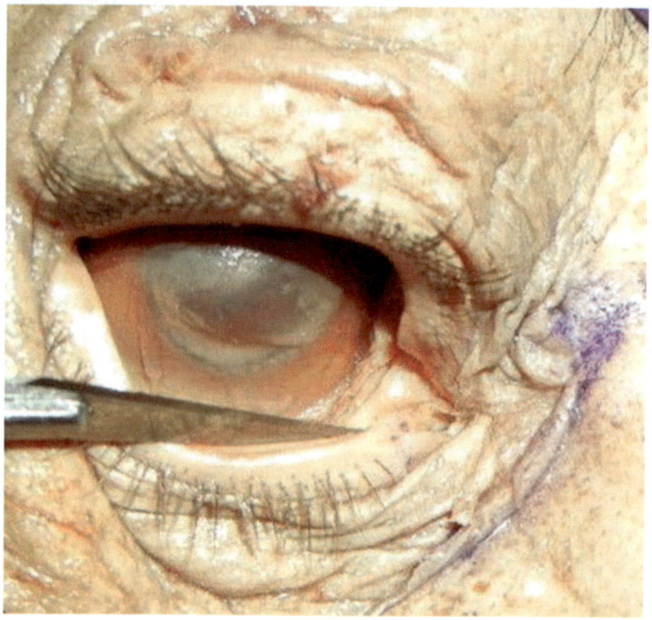

Fig. 7.29 #11 blade in punctum to "unroof" the canaliculus

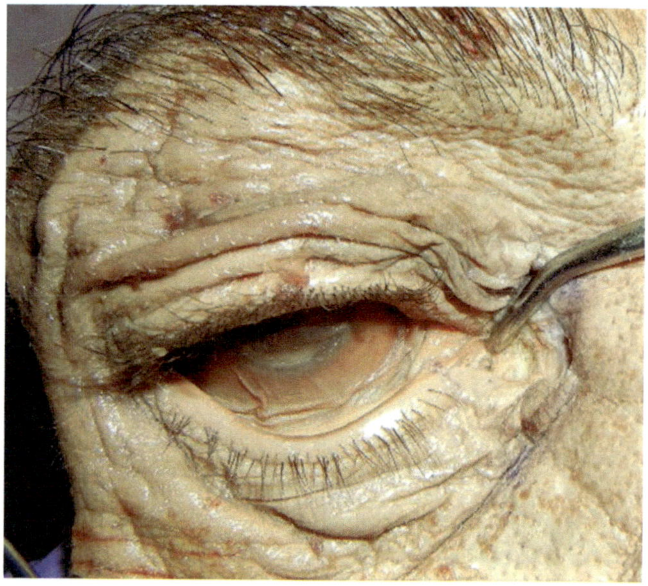

Fig. 7.30 Common internal punctum

17. With a #11 blade, vertically incise the eyelid margin at the punctum (Fig. 7.27) to demonstrate the vertical canaliculus and canalicular ampulla.
18. Attempt to pass a probe through the canaliculus into the sac (Fig. 7.28).
19. With a #11 blade, "unroof" the canaliculus (Fig. 7.29), and demonstrate the common internal punctum (Fig. 7.30).

Clinical correlation: A canaliculotomy of the horizontal canaliculus is often necessary for the treatment and removal of canaliculothiasis.

20. Next, place a pointer in the bony nasolacrimal fossa (Fig. 7.31), and push through the bone confirming its exit in the region of the middle meatus, anterior to the middle turbinate (Fig. 7.32).

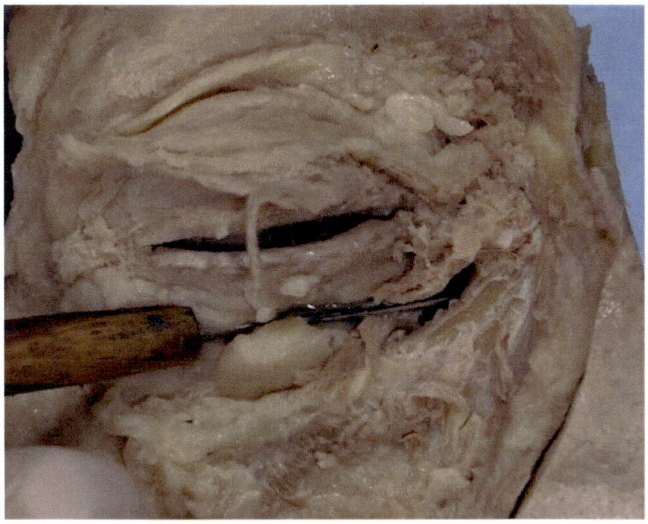

Fig. 7.31 Probe in the bony lacrimal fossa

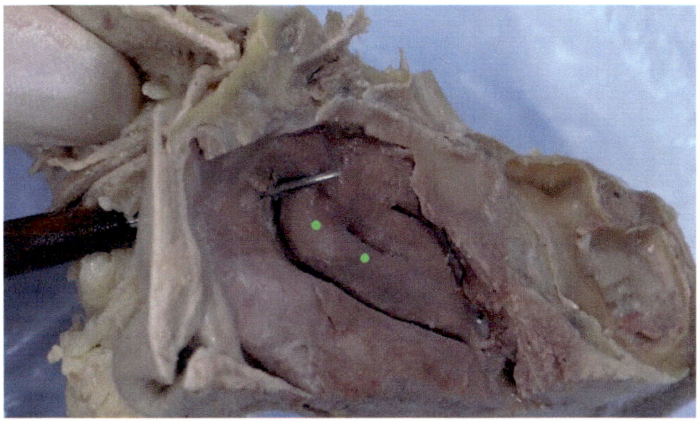

Fig. 7.32 Probe exiting in the region of the middle meatus, anterior to the middle turbinate (green dots)

Clinical correlation: Appreciation of this three-dimensional anatomy is important when performing dacryocystorhinostomy (DCR) surgery, as this is the site of entrance into the nose from the bony lacrimal fossa. Occasionally, an anterior middle turbinectomy needs to be performed to prevent obstruction of the dacryocystorhinostomy by a large middle turbinate.

21. Place the pointer down the bony nasolacrimal canal (Fig. 7.33), confirming its exit under the inferior turbinate (Fig. 7.34). Note its inferior, posterior, and slightly lateral course from the lacrimal sac fossa. Its slightly lateral course is variable depending on individual bone features. In Fig. 7.33, the direction is inferior, posterior and slightly medial.

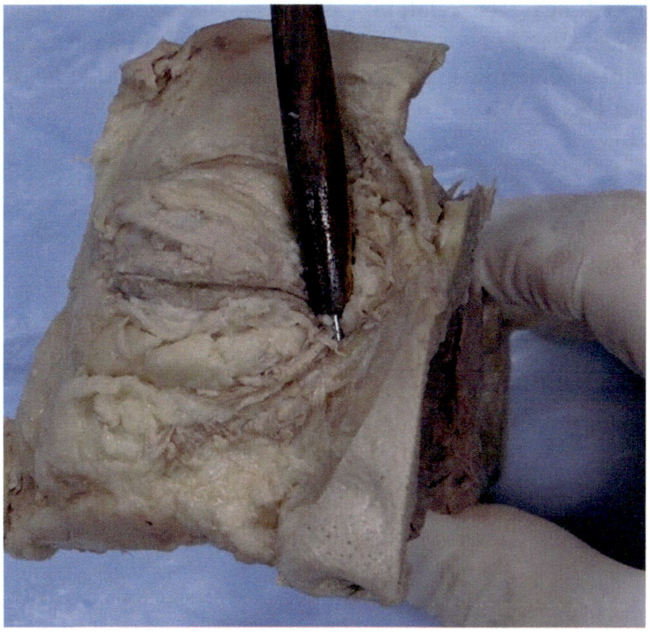

Fig. 7.33 Probe in bony nasolacrimal canal

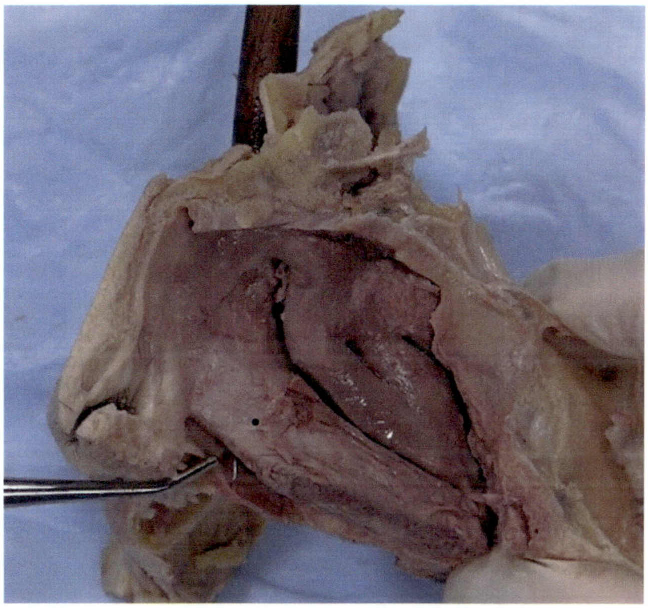

Fig. 7.34 Probe (at tip of pointer) seen exiting under the inferior turbinate (black dot)

Clinical correlation: Appreciation of this three-dimensional anatomy is important when identifying lacrimal probes or retrieving lacrimal intubation tubes in pediatric patients.

Suggested Reading

Beard C, Quickert M. Anatomy of the orbit. second ed. Birmingham, AL: Aesculapius Publishing Company; 1977. p. 15–7.

Bedrossian EH Jr. The lacrimal system. In: Tasman W, Jaeger E, editors. Foundations of clinical ophthalmology, vol. 1. Philadelphia: Lippincott; 1996. p. 1–16.

Jones LT. Anatomy of the tear system. Int Ophthalmol Clin. 1973;13:3.

Jones LT, Wobig JL. Surgery of the eyelids and lacrimal system. Birmingham, AL: Aesculapius Publishing; 1976. p. 7–9. 67-70

Tanenbaum M, McCord C Jr. Lacrimal drainage system. In: Tasman W, Jaeger EA, editors. Duane's ophthalmology, Vol. 4. Philadelphia: Lippincott Williams & Wilkins; 2007.

Index

E. H. Bedrossian, Jr et al. (eds.), *Anatomy of the Eyelid, Orbit, and Lacrimal System*,
https://doi.org/10.1007/978-3-030-88265-5

GPSR Compliance

The European Union's (EU) General Product Safety Regulation (GPSR) is a set of rules that requires consumer products to be safe and our obligations to ensure this.

If you have any concerns about our products, you can contact us on ProductSafety@springernature.com

In case Publisher is established outside the EU, the EU authorized representative is:

Springer Nature Customer Service Center GmbH
Europaplatz 3
69115 Heidelberg, Germany

Batch number: 10731530

Printed by Printforce, the Netherlands